The Glycemic Index Diet and Cookbook

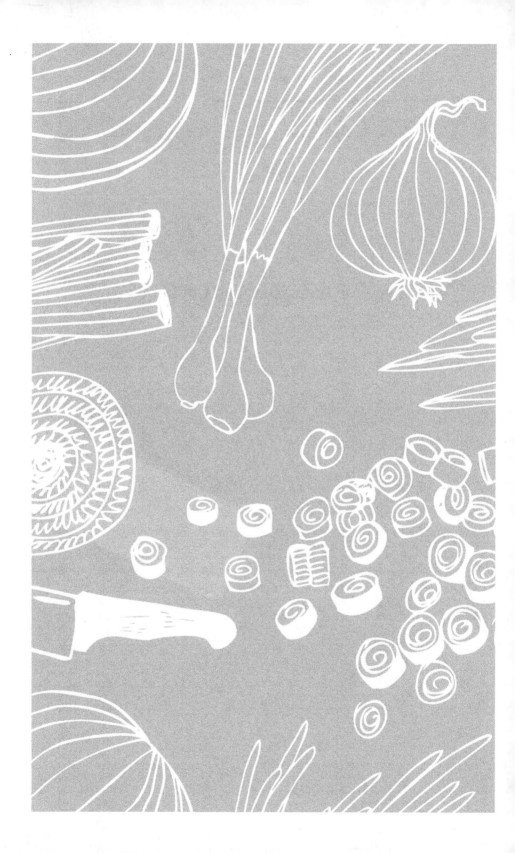

The Glycemic Index

Diet and Cookbook

RECIPES TO CHART GLYCEMIC INDEX LOAD AND LOSE WEIGHT

HEALDSBURG PRESS

For general information on our other products and services or to obtain technical support, please contact our Customer Care Department within the United States at (866) 744-2665, or outside the United States at (510) 253-0500.

Healdsburg Press publishes its books in a variety of electronic and print formats. Some content that appears in print may not be available in electronic books, and vice versa.

ISBN: Print 978-1-62315-246-8 | eBook 978-1-62315-329-8

Contents

Introduction

You've probably heard of the glycemic index in the media or at your health provider's office. You may have come across it while searching for information on how to eat better and reduce your blood sugar. If you have diabetes—or fear you are at risk for developing diabetes—your doctor has likely advised you to reduce the amount of sugar in your diet. Or maybe you're just looking for a simple way to eat healthy and lose or maintain your weight. If any of these describe you, this book is an excellent resource.

The Glycemic Index Diet and Cookbook is intended to help you monitor and control the level of sugar in your diet. In this book, you'll find essential information to better understand the glycemic index and to make appropriate changes in your eating habits.

The glycemic index (GI) is a measure of how fast a given food causes a rise in blood sugar. Foods are scored on a range from 0 to 100; foods with higher GI scores cause blood sugar levels to rise faster than foods with lower scores. Why is this important? Not only can high blood sugar levels lead to unhealthy weight gain, but if your blood sugar levels are high for long periods of time, you may be at greater risk of developing other health problems, such as heart disease and some types of cancer.

This book is a handbook and cookbook all in one. Part One introduces the Glycemic Index Diet and the basic science behind it, including the effects of diet on blood glucose as well as the effects of blood glucose on health. This section explains how the glycemic index can inform your diet, including quick reference charts that show the GI scores of various foods. Becoming familiar with where certain foods fall on the glycemic index can help you make better eating choices—whether you're cooking at home or dining out. A 14-day meal plan offers two weeks' worth of healthy suggestions for breakfast, lunch, dinner, and snacks.

The more than 75 recipes in Part Two will help you plan and make meals that are delicious and have optimal glycemic index values. Including recipes for every meal of the day—and incorporating foods that are accessible and flavorful—these recipes are tasty, healthy, and easy to prepare!

Use the handbook and cookbook features in tandem to launch yourself on the path toward achieving your health goals. Consult Part One to familiarize yourself with what the glycemic index is and how it works. Meanwhile, try out some of the recipes featured in Part Two and start eating healthier right away! Return to the earlier chapters anytime you want a quick review of the glycemic index, and flip to the food charts or meal plan as handy references while making your weekly shopping list or creating your own healthy variation of the two-week meal plan.

Welcome to the Glycemic Index Diet, and cheers to your better health!

PART ONE

The Glycemic Index Diet

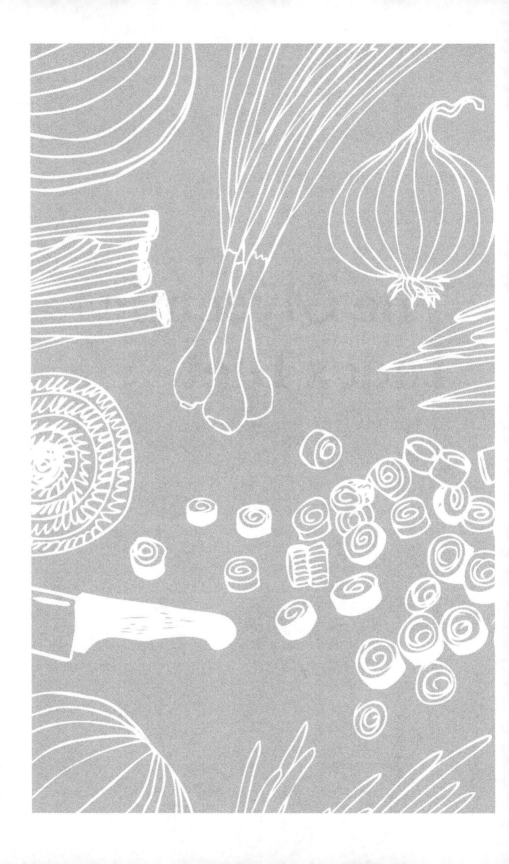

CHAPTER 1

Blood Glucose and Your Health

WHAT IS BLOOD GLUCOSE?

Blood glucose is the medical term for sugar in the bloodstream. Blood sugar is an important source of energy for the cells in your body, and having the right blood glucose level helps your cells function well. "Blood glucose level" is just another way of saying "blood sugar level," meaning the amount of sugar in your blood.

There are two ways that sugar can enter your bloodstream: through what you eat and from sugar stores found in your liver. Carbohydrates are found in the foods that you eat. When your body digests food, it breaks carbohydrates down into glucose (sugar). So if you eat foods containing a lot of carbohydrates, especially certain types of carbohydrates called "simple carbohydrates," you're more likely to increase your blood glucose levels.

Your body breaks down and absorbs simple carbohydrates more quickly than complex carbohydrates, so eating simple carbohydrates causes your blood glucose levels to rise quickly. Complex carbohydrates are healthier for you, because your body breaks them down more slowly, keeping your blood glucose levels more stable. Complex carbohydrates (also known as "slow carbs") also stay in your digestive tract longer than simple carbs and thus keep you feeling full longer. In Chapter 2, you'll find a list of common food sources of complex and simple carbohydrates as well as specific foods that will aid you in lowering your blood glucose levels.

Don't worry: You can still eat carbohydrates while following the Glycemic Index Diet. If you can't bear to give up bread, for example, you can eat whole-wheat bread (in moderation). You will need to minimize your intake of processed foods, such as frozen waffles and pancakes made from boxed mixes, because they can increase your blood glucose levels. While fruits and vegetables contain carbohydrates, you can eat large amounts of both, although some fruits and vegetables are better for you than others. For instance, you should avoid potatoes, which rank relatively high on the glycemic index, but you can eat lots of low-GI broccoli and spinach.

Many hormones help your body regulate its blood sugar levels, but the primary ones are insulin and glucagon. When your blood sugar is high (because you've eaten a high-GI food), your body releases insulin, which helps the sugar in your blood enter cells so they can use it as energy. When your blood sugar is low, your body releases glucagon, which releases sugar that's stored in your liver into your bloodstream. Ongoing imbalances in your blood sugar can affect your health. Over time, if blood sugar levels stay high or cycle rapidly, your body will have trouble responding to insulin. This can lead to health problems such as type 2 diabetes, obesity, high blood pressure, stroke, and heart disease. The goal of the Glycemic Index Diet is to help you make wise eating choices that will keep your blood sugar levels balanced.

HOW DOES BLOOD GLUCOSE AFFECT YOUR HEALTH?

As mentioned above, health care professionals have determined that blood glucose levels can affect your long-term health. Regularly eating foods with high glycemic index scores puts you at a greater risk of developing health conditions such as heart disease, cancer, diabetes, and dementia. Conversely, controlling your blood glucose levels by eating a low-GI diet can help reduce your risk of these and other ailments and enhance your overall health.

Stay Heart Healthy

You can protect your heart health by eating a low-GI diet. In a ten-year study of more than 75,000 women, researchers found that eating foods with high glycemic index scores increased the chances that a woman would develop heart disease. (This was independent of other factors that might increase such risk.) Another study, based on dietary questionnaires of more than 47,000 Italian adults, showed that among female respondents, the 25 percent who consumed the most carbohydrates overall had approximately twice the risk of heart disease as the 25 percent who consumed the least. When the carbs were separated into high- and low-GI categories, increased intake of high-GI foods was significantly associated with greater risk of coronary heart disease, and low-GI carbs were not.

Another study looked at the relationship between diet and blood lipids in young people, and found that the higher the youths' glycemic load (derived from foods' glycemic index scores *and* their total carbohydrates), the lower their levels of HDL cholesterol. Often termed "good" cholesterol, HDL helps clean your arteries of LDL or "bad" cholesterol and reduces your risk of heart disease. Conversely, several studies have shown that foods with lower glycemic index scores may increase HDL cholesterol. So you may very well improve your heart health by eating a low-GI diet.

Reduce Cancer Risk

Studies show that eating higher-GI foods may increase the risk of several types of cancer. For example, large studies conducted in the United States and Italy found that people who ate foods with high glycemic index scores were more likely to be diagnosed with colon cancer—the second most common cause of cancer-related deaths in the United States—than individuals who ate foods with low glycemic index scores. A federally funded 2012 study by the Dana-Farber Cancer Institute in Boston found that among patients with advanced colon cancer, those who had the highest glycemic load and carbohydrate intake were nearly twice as likely to see their cancer return.

If you are female, eating foods with low GI scores may help reduce your risk of breast cancer. One study showed that women who, during their annual breast exams, were found to have areas of high-density breast tissue—which makes it harder to interpret a mammogram—were more likely to have diets with a high glycemic index score. Another study, of Italian women, determined that having a high concentration of carbohydrates from high-GI foods was associated with greater breast cancer risk.

Manage or Avoid Diabetes

Studies have shown that people who eat a high-GI diet are at a higher risk of developing type 2 diabetes. Because high-GI foods significantly increase blood glucose levels, they also increase the body's demand for insulin. This can cause, or contribute to, problems with the pancreas (which produces insulin) and this in turn may eventually lead to diabetes. Also, by increasing the production of fatty acids after meals, high-GI foods can decrease the body's response to insulin. High-GI foods cause rapid spikes in blood sugar levels and so can worsen diabetes symptoms, whereas studies have shown that a low-GI diet can help you better control the disease by keeping blood sugar levels more stable.

For most people with diabetes, balancing total carbohydrate intake with physical activity and insulin or other medications is key to managing blood glucose levels. But because the *type* of carbohydrates you consume affects blood glucose levels, using glycemic index scores can help you fine-tune your blood glucose management.

If you don't have diabetes but have been told by your health provider that you have metabolic syndrome, referring to a group of risk factors that jointly raise your risk of heart disease and other health problems including diabetes, eating a low-GI diet may help you control the symptoms. Type 2 diabetes doesn't develop from eating carbs, but rather from being overweight. If you are somewhat overweight, eating a low-GI diet is a good way to get on track toward your weight-loss goal. If you are obese, eating a low-GI diet will help you lose weight and avoid the spikes in blood sugar that can lead to glucose intolerance and diabetes. (Glucose intolerance occurs when the body does not respond properly to blood sugar levels—specifically, it doesn't produce enough insulin— or the insulin that it produces isn't able to get sugar that's in the bloodstream into cells so that they can use it as energy.)

Feed Your Brain

Where the majority of fats in your diet come from does matter. Studies have found that diets reliant on fats from fish, vegetable oils, nonstarchy vegetables, and low-GI fruits were associated with a lower risk of Alzheimer's disease. Furthermore, in populations that ate these foods, there was a slower decline from mild cognitive impairment to Alzheimer's disease.

A study published in the *New England Journal of Medicine* found that people without diabetes who had higher average glucose levels had an 18 percent greater risk of developing dementia than people with lower average glucose levels. People *with* diabetes had a 40 percent greater risk of developing dementia if their glucose levels were higher on average than people who kept their blood glucose levels lower. After fasting for eight hours, a blood glucose level between 70 and 100 mg/dL (measurement in milligrams per deciliter of blood) is generally considered a normal test result.

Perhaps most exciting is a 2011 nutritional study of 49 adults whose average age was 69. This study was unique in that, instead of focusing on one single food or nutrient, the VA Puget Sound researchers who conducted it looked at participants' *whole* diet. For four weeks, researchers carefully measured, analyzed, and delivered food to the participants. The low-GI diet consisted of 25 percent fat (of which less than 7 percent was saturated fat), 55 to 60 percent low-GI carbs (those with a glycemic index score of less than 55), and 15 to 20 percent protein. The high-GI diet consisted of 45 percent fat (25 percent of which was saturated fat), 35 to 40 percent high-GI carbs (those with a glycemic index of greater than 70), and 15 to 20 percent protein.

The researchers found that the low-GI diet not only lowered the levels of substances found in the participants' cerebrospinal fluid that are associated with the development of Alzheimer's, but it also improved participants' scores on a memory test. All this in only four weeks! The encouraging outcome of this study shows that a diet with lots of low-GI foods can lower your likelihood of developing Alzheimer's.

Improve Overall Health

Historically, in many cultures outside of the United States, eating low-GI foods was natural. When peoples such as the Pima Indians of South America and the Aborigines in Australia adopted Western habits and began eating a lot of high-GI foods, diabetes was an all-too-common outcome.

The Glycemic Index Diet encourages you to make thoughtful choices about the foods you put into your body. Committing to a low-GI eating plan can have a positive impact on many areas of your health, ranging from protecting your vision health to achieving and maintain your ideal weight. The following health issues are attributable to GI levels in your diet.

Constipation: If you eat low-GI foods, your diet will have lots of fiber in it, which helps keep you regular. For example, low-GI fruits and vegetables are loaded with fiber. If you often experience constipation, some studies have suggested that your symptoms will improve if you consistently eat a low-GI diet.

Hypoglycemia: The official term for low blood sugar, hypoglycemia is a problem for diabetics, who can also have blood sugar levels that are too *high*. When you eat a low-GI diet, your body is better able to control your blood sugar levels because they don't rise or fall quickly. The foods recommended in this book help keep your blood sugar levels even, helping to avoid extremes in your blood sugar levels, which can be a serious problem if you're diabetic.

Polycystic Ovarian Syndrome (PCOS): If you are a woman who suffers from polycystic ovarian syndrome, you are aware of the difficulties of this condition. Many women with PCOS suffer from insulin resistance that is similar to diabetes, and some develop type 2 diabetes. If you have PCOS and are overweight, you understand how difficult it is to lose weight with this condition. A low-GI diet may help you lose weight, control your blood sugar levels, and control your PCOS symptoms.

Age-related macular degeneration (AMD): The primary cause of irreversible blindness, AMD appears to share several carbohydrate-related risk factors with diabetes and associated diseases, and a study published in the *American Journal of Clinical Nutrition* found that AMD is 42 percent higher among people with a high-GI diet. According to the study, eating a lower-GI diet would eliminate 20 percent of AMD cases.

Syndrome X: A high intake of carbohydrates has been reported to produce higher insulin levels in your body. In turn, it's possible that repeatedly stimulating your body to produce high amounts of insulin can hasten an age-related decline in insulin secretion, potentially leading to what is known as non-insulin-dependent diabetes mellitus (NIDDM) as well as a host of other medical conditions jointly known as Syndrome X: hypertriglyceridemia, which is associated with increased risk of cardiovascular illness and acute pancreatitis; increased LDL (bad) cholesterol; decreased HDL (good) cholesterol; abnormally high blood pressure, referred to as hypertension; hyperuricemia, or too much uric acid in the blood; and obesity. Multiple studies suggest that high-GI carbs contribute to chronic hyperinsulinemia, or excess levels of insulin circulating in the blood. Overall, there is a clear correlation between excessive intake of high-GI carbs and the development of insulin resistance and its subsequent disorders. Inversely, eating a low-GI diet has been clearly shown to help treat and prevent chronic diseases.

Overeating: Studies have linked high-GI foods with overeating. One study found that the higher the glycemic index score of the diet, the less satiated the participants were and the higher their insulin levels. Another study found that the behavior of additional eating was 53 percent more likely after a high-GI meal than after a medium-GI meal and 81 percent greater than after a low-GI meal. The authors concluded that high-GI meals promote excessive food intake in obese individuals.

Following the Glycemic Index Diet is a wonderful way to lose weight. Studies have shown that when you eat a low-GI diet, you burn more calories at rest than if you eat a regular low-fat diet. Adding regular exercise to your weight-loss regimen will achieve even better results. A large European study found that a high-protein, reduced-GI diet increased the ability of overweight individuals to lose weight and maintain their weight loss over time. If you use the glycemic index guidelines in this book to make your food choices, you may be more likely to reach and stay at your ideal weight.

When you eat foods that have a low glycemic index score, you feel full longer. As a result, you will likely eat less often, which will help decrease your calorie intake along with maintaining a more balanced blood sugar level and promoting overall health.

Exercise

Along with your diet, exercise is important for maintaining your overall health. If you want to lose weight, exercise is an essential part of an overall weight-loss plan.

Each pound of fat that you need to lose contains 3,500 calories. So if you want to change your weight, the best and most proven system is to eat less and exercise more. Even if weight loss isn't one of your goals, exercise can improve your mood and overall fitness. Plus, exercise will simply help you feel better!

INTERPRETING THE GLYCEMIC INDEX DIET RESPONSIBLY

Although you can expect healthful results by following the Glycemic Index Diet, it is important to keep in mind that no diet is perfect. Studies have shown mixed levels of satisfaction and results with the Glycemic Index Diet. Critics note that, in this diet, foods are ranked solely by their glycemic index scores, and that low-GI foods can in fact be high in fat and calories.

It's true that the Glycemic Index Diet ranks foods based on their glucose levels without regard to other factors that may affect their overall nutritional value. This diet doesn't limit the *types* of foods that you can choose, it just limits you to low-GI foods. You should always use good judgment in making choices, as some foods with lower GI scores can be less healthy than foods with higher GI scores. For example, some fats are good for you, whereas other fats are unhealthy. You can find good fats in nuts, olives, and salmon, and bad fats in regular cheese and pork. So if you decide to choose lots of low-GI foods that are also high in calories, sugar, and saturated fats, you could develop some of the same health problems that this diet aims to prevent.

In other words, don't try to cheat the system. As long as you use common sense and work toward a healthy overall diet, using glycemic index numbers to guide your food choices will enhance your overall health and provide a powerful tool for weight loss and maintenance as well as blood glucose management.

SIGNS YOUR BLOOD GLUCOSE LEVEL IS TOO HIGH

High blood sugar (aka hyperglycemia) is a serious health problem. There are two types of symptoms that you should look for to know whether you suffer from this condition. If you eat a lot of sugary foods but have not been diagnosed with diabetes, you may experience the following symptoms when your blood sugar levels are high:

- Thirst
- Frequent illness
- Fatigue
- Yeast infections (vaginal yeast infections, rashes in the groin area and other moist areas of the body not due to psoriasis, or athlete's foot)
- Frequent hunger

If you experience these symptoms often, you should consult a health practitioner. Fortunately, you can relieve these symptoms by controlling your blood sugar and by eating a diet of low-GI foods.

More serious symptoms, which can also be caused by high blood sugar levels, are blurry vision, confusion, or stroke symptoms. If experiencing any of these, you should see a health professional *immediately*.

It's possible to measure your blood glucose, at the doctor's office or even at a home. If you are diabetic, you are likely familiar with this process. But if you aren't diabetic and aren't experiencing the symptoms described above, you don't need to go to the extreme of drawing blood to determine your blood glucose level unless your health provider advises it.

Instead, you can set out to reduce and stabilize your blood glucose level with a low-GI diet by eating the foods listed in the next chapter. Think of your blood glucose level like a landscape you have the potential to help create: Over the course of a given day, you want the spikes in your blood sugar levels to look less like a mountain range, with severe peaks and valleys, and more like rolling hills, with only gradual ups and downs.

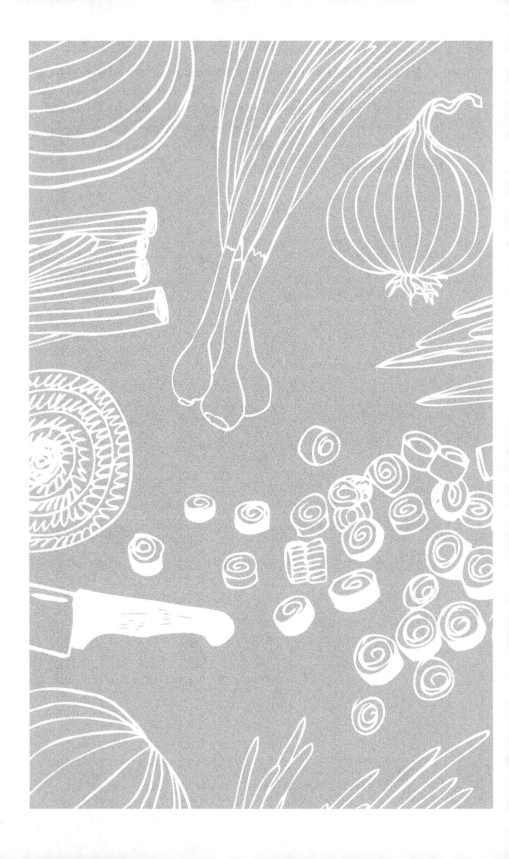

CHAPTER 2

Starting the Glycemic Index Diet

This chapter provides information on common foods that have high or low glycemic index scores. It's intended to start you thinking about your diet and considering how you can make changes or replacements that will result in a lower overall blood glucose level.

A food's glycemic index score is an indication of how much that food will increase your blood sugar if you eat it. As mentioned in the previous chapter, the term "glycemic load" refers to the food's glycemic index score *and* its total carbohydrates. Knowing a food's glycemic load can help you predict how much your blood sugar will increase if you eat that food, and how much insulin your body will produce. However, don't get bogged down in the specifics of the glycemic index and glycemic load numbers of every food. It's impractical to check these numbers for all the foods you eat. Instead, focus on your *overall* diet. If your overall glycemic load is low, then having an occasional sweet treat isn't a problem. If you eat one high-GI food combined with several low-GI foods, then the total glycemic load of your meal or snack will be lower. If there are certain high-GI foods you can't bring yourself to give up, learn to combine them with low-GI foods to balance out the meal. Rather than obsessing about each food's specific glycemic index or glycemic load number, focus on maintaining a healthy overall eating pattern with a low overall glycemic load.

GENERAL GI GUIDELINES

Fiber and fat tend to lower a food's glycemic index score. Fiber is an important carbohydrate found in many foods, but it doesn't change blood glucose levels when you eat it. That's because fiber isn't digested by your body; it passes through your digestive track undigested and can help you feel full. So if you eat high-fiber foods, you will feel full, eat less, and be more likely to lose weight.

Eating fat makes your body digest food more slowly, and foods with fats in them have a lower glycemic index score. This doesn't mean that you should simply add fat to your diet, however! You should focus on *good* fats, which are detailed later in this chapter. Proteins are another important part of the Glycemic Index Diet. Research suggests that, like fiber, protein also helps keep you feeling full and can help you lose weight while eating a low-GI diet. Other factors can affect a food's glycemic index, such as the following:

- *Ripeness:* The riper a fruit or vegetable is, the higher its GI.
- *Processing:* Juice has a higher GI than whole fruit, and mashed potatoes have a higher GI than baked potatoes.
- *Cooking method/time:* Pasta cooked al dente has a lower GI than soft-cooked pasta.

Remember, too, that regardless of a food's glycemic index score, keeping an eye on portion sizes is important for managing blood glucose levels and for losing (or maintaining) weight. Also, as mentioned earlier, many nutritious foods have a higher glycemic index score than foods with less nutritional value; for example, oatmeal has a higher score than chocolate. Using foods' GI scores as a guide for healthy eating needs to be balanced with the basic nutrition principles of variety and moderation—and a healthy dose of common sense.

Counting Carbs

If you have diabetes, you may be accustomed to counting carbs, and you may be wondering if keeping track of GI is a better strategy. In that case, the glycemic index scale is intended as an *additional* resource, not a replacement for your current technique. The glycemic index scale was first developed to help diabetics better control their blood sugar levels. It is now also used to help people who have been told that they have prediabetes (aka metabolic syndrome) as well as people without diabetes who wish to control their blood sugar levels. The glycemic index scale has helped people lose weight and improve their health without going on a strict diet.

Keep in mind that using the glycemic index scale alone to help you choose foods will not result in a true low-carb diet, because doing so doesn't involve counting carbs. However, a food's glycemic load is determined by figuring out the amount of carbohydrates in each serving, multiplying that figure by the food's glycemic index score, and then dividing that number by 100. Carbohydrates are taken into consideration when determining a food's glycemic load, but they aren't the sole focus. (See Chapter 4 for glycemic load values of common foods.)

There's no one diet or system that works for everyone with diabetes. The important thing is to tailor a healthful meal plan to your personal preferences and lifestyle, which in turn will help you achieve your goals for blood glucose, cholesterol, and triglyceride levels as well as blood pressure and weight management.

UNDERSTANDING SIMPLE AND COMPLEX CARBOHYDRATES

The types of foods you eat directly affect your blood glucose levels. All foods contain carbohydrates, but some have more than others. Your body digests simple carbohydrates more quickly than complex carbs, and turns simple carbs into sugar in the bloodstream.

Simple Carbohydrates

When you eat food that's filled with simple carbs, your blood sugar levels increase much faster than when you eat foods with complex carbohydrates. The following are four common sources of simple carbs. (These tables aren't comprehensive listings of all simple carb–rich foods, but they'll give you a good sense of high- and low-GI foods.)

1. White flour and products made with white flour
White flour is a major ingredient in breads, cakes, and pasta. Products made with white flour are the most common source of simple carbohydrates after simple sugars, and are among the highest on the glycemic index. An alternative to white flour is whole-wheat flour. However, keep in mind that if you choose whole-wheat products, you may not decrease your glycemic index score as much as you would if you avoided flour products altogether. And always check nutritional labels; some brands may have more sugar than others and even some varieties within brands may have higher GI numbers.

High-GI Products Made with White Flour	Lower-GI Alternatives
Breads	**Breads**
Breadsticks (white)	Bran bread
English muffins (white)	Breadsticks (whole-wheat)
Flour tortillas (white)	Corn tortillas
French or Italian bread	Lavash (whole-wheat)
Lavash or roll-ups (white)	English muffins (whole-wheat)
Matzoh (plain)	Matzoh (whole-wheat)
Pita (white)	Oatmeal bread
Sourdough bread	Pita (whole-wheat)
White bread	Pumpernickel bread
	Rye bread
Cereals	Whole-grain bread
Cream of Rice	Whole-wheat bread
Cream of Wheat	
Grape Nuts	**Cereals**
Kashi 7 Whole Grain Nuggets	Kashi 7 Whole Grain Puffs
Shredded Wheat	Steel-cut oats
Special K	Total Protein
Total Whole Grain	Wheat bran (raw)
Wheatena	Wheat germ (toasted)

2. Sweeteners

Corn syrup, high-fructose corn syrup, and sugar are in lots of foods, and all of these sweeteners are simple carbohydrates. Natural sweeteners such as honey, maple syrup, and molasses—though healthier—are simple carbohydrates, too.

High-GI Sweeteners	Lower-GI Alternatives
Brown sugar	Batey Natural Light (stevia and turbinado sugar)
Corn syrup	Fructevia (fructose and stevia)
Honey	Ideal (xylitol and sucralose)
Molasses	NatraTaste Gold (sucralose)
Pancake	Nature Sweet Crystals (maltitol)
syrup	Nature Sweet Brown Crystals (maltitol)
Maple syrup	Pure Via (stevia)
White sugar	Splenda (sucralose)
	Splenda Sugar Blend (sucralose and white sugar)
	SweetLeaf (stevia)
	Truvia (stevia)
	Whey Low (fructose and other sugars)
	Xylitol
	Zsweet (erythritol)

3. Beverages

Your best beverage choice is always water—still or carbonated—which is 100 percent carb-free.

In small amounts, fruit juice can be nutritious. However, many juices are high on the glycemic index scale (meaning they increase your blood sugar quickly) and can be a major source of sugar in your diet. Not all juices are equal: Some are lower on the glycemic index scale than others. In order to make wise choices, become familiar with particular juices' glycemic index scores.

Sodas are full of sugar and are a major source of simple carbohydrates in many Americans' diets. Drinking soda is believed to be a major cause of obesity in the United States.

While some alcohols, such as light beer and wine, have low GI numbers, it's important to drink in moderation if choosing alcohol—and avoid it altogether when taking certain medications.

High-GI Beverages	Lower-GI Alternatives
Fruit Juices	**Alcohol**
Apple juice (unsweetened)	Cocktails containing soda or fruit juice
Apricot nectar	**Fruit Juices**
Cranberry juice cocktail (regular)	Cranberry juice cocktail (light)
Fruit punch	Grapefruit juice (unsweetened)
Grape juice (unsweetened)	Lemon juice
Grapefruit juice (sweetened)	Lime juice
Guava nectar	Carrot juice
Mango nectar	Sugar-free powdered juice (such as Minute Maid Light, Crystal Light, or Kool-Aid Sugar Free)
Orange juice; orange juice blends	Tomato juice
Passion fruit (fresh)	Vegetable juice cocktail (such as V8)
Peach nectar	Water (still or sparkling)
Pear nectar	
Pineapple juice	**Other Beverages**
Prune juice	Coffee (unsweetened)
	Tea
	Diet energy drinks
	Diet sodas
Other Beverages	
Cola and cherry cola	**(in moderation if at all)**
Energy drinks (regular)	Beer, light or low-carb
Ginger ale	Bourbon
Grape soda	Champagne
Root beer/birch beer	Gin
Sweetened tea	Rum
Tonic water	Scotch
	Vodka
	Wine, red or white

4. Fruits and vegetables

Of course fruits and vegetables are good for you, but some are a source of simple carbs and thus have a high glycemic index score. The following table gives you a sense of which is which, so you can choose many flavorful alternatives for your daily menus and save the higher-GI ones for a treat now and then. Fresh or unsweetened frozen fruit is best; in general, avoid buying any fruit canned in syrup, and any sweetened dried or frozen fruit.

High-GI Fruits	Lower-GI Alternatives
Apples (dried or in applesauce)	Apples (fresh)
Apricots (canned in syrup/ juice)	Apricots (fresh)
	Blackberries (fresh or frozen)
Bananas (fresh or dried)	Blueberries (fresh or frozen)
Cherries, sour (fresh)	Cherries, sweet (fresh, dried, or frozen)
Dates (fresh or dried)	Clementines (fresh)
Fruit cocktail (canned in syrup/juice/water)	Coconut (fresh or unsweetened shredded)
Grapes/raisins (dried)	Cranberries (fresh, dried, or in cranberry sauce)
Mangoes (dried or frozen)	
Nectarines (fresh)	Figs (fresh or dried)
Oranges (fresh or canned in juice)	Grapefruit (fresh or canned in juice)
	Grapes (fresh)
Papaya (dried)	Kiwi (fresh)
Peaches (dried or canned in syrup/juice)	Mangoes (fresh)
	Melons (fresh)
Pears (fresh or canned in syrup/juice)	Papaya (fresh or frozen)
	Peaches (fresh or canned in water)
Pineapple (dried or canned in syrup/juice)	Pears (canned in water)
	Persimmons (fresh)
Plantains (fresh or dried)	Pineapple (fresh or canned in water)
Plums/prunes (dried)	Plums (fresh)
Strawberries (fresh, dried, or frozen)	Pomegranates (fresh)
	Raspberries (fresh or frozen)
Watermelon (fresh)	Tangerines (fresh)

High-GI Vegetables	Lower-GI Vegetables
Beets	Note: *Many vegetables have low GI*
Carrots	*numbers. See page 24 for a list of*
Parsnips	*common low-GI vegetables.*
Potatoes (white)	
Pumpkins	
Rutabaga	
Sweet potatoes	

Complex Carbohydrates

Complex carbohydrates are more difficult for the body to break down and so do not increase your blood sugar levels as quickly as simple carbs do. The following are four examples of complex carbohydrates.

1. Whole grains
Grains such as wheat, barley, and oats are high in complex carbs and fiber. Breads made from these grains are lower on the glycemic index scale than breads made with white flour, although you're likely to find some amount of simple carbs in any bread product. So always use common sense and make a practice of eating moderate amounts of these foods.

Low-GI Whole Grains

Amaranth	Quinoa
Barley	Rye
Brown rice	Sorghum
Buckwheat	Spelt
Bulgur	Teff
Farro	Whole wheat
Millet	Wild rice
Oats	

2. Nuts, seeds, and legumes
Nuts, seeds, and legumes are excellent sources of fiber and protein. In addition, many of these foods, such as lentils, are vitamin-packed. Foods in this category are also high in complex carbs.

Low-GI Nuts, Seeds, and Legumes

Almonds

Black beans

Brazil nuts

Cannellini beans

Cashews

Chickpeas

Edamame

Fava beans

Green beans

Hazelnuts (filberts)

Kidney beans

Lentils (green, red, yellow)

Lima beans

Mung beans

Peanuts

Peas (black-eyed, green, split)

Pine nuts

Pinto beans

Pistachios

Pumpkin seeds

Sesame seeds

Soybeans

Sunflower seeds

Walnuts

3. Dairy products

Dairy products are a good source of complex carbohydrates, and many low-fat dairy products are also low on the glycemic index scale. However, remember that low-fat and fat-free products can have high calorie content and more sugar than you want to eat. When considering reduced-fat, low-fat, and fat-free options, it's a good idea to read nutritional labels carefully and be wary of sugar, flour, thickeners, and salt that may be added to the products, as well as the amount of cholesterol. Balance low-fat choices with foods that contain "good" or naturally occurring fats (see page 25 for an explanation of good fats and food sources).

Low-GI Dairy Products

Low-fat ice cream

Low-fat sour cream

Low-fat yogurt (fresh or frozen)

Nonfat milk

Reduced-fat cheese

4. Fruits and vegetables

Since some fruits and vegetables can be sources of simple carbs, familiarizing yourself with the ones that rank lower on the glycemic index will help you make wise (not to mention delicious) choices. Onions and tomatoes are high in vitamins and in complex carbs. Potatoes rank relatively high on the glycemic index, so save them for special-occasion meals. Have fun trying low-GI fruits and veggies you may not have tasted before!

Low-GI Fruits

Apples (fresh)
Apricots (fresh)
Blackberries (fresh or frozen)
Blueberries (fresh or frozen)
Cherries, sweet (fresh, dried or frozen)
Clementines (fresh)
Coconut (fresh or unsweetened shredded)
Cranberries (fresh, dried, or in cranberry sauce)
Figs (fresh or dried)
Grapefruit (fresh or canned in juice)
Grapes (fresh)

Guava (fresh)
Kiwi (fresh)
Mangoes (fresh)
Melons (fresh)
Papayas (fresh or frozen)
Peaches (fresh or canned in water)
Pears (canned in water)
Persimmons (fresh)
Pineapples (fresh or canned in water)
Plums (fresh)
Pomegranates (fresh)
Raspberries (fresh or frozen)
Tangerines (fresh)

Low-GI Vegetables

Artichoke
Asparagus
Bean sprouts
Beet greens
Bell pepper
Broccoli
Brussels sprouts
Cabbage
Carrot
Cauliflower
Celery
Chiles

Cucumber
Eggplant
Green beans
Green peas
Lettuce
Mushrooms
Mustard greens
Onions
Radishes
Spinach
Swiss chard
Tomatoes

Keep in mind that carbohydrates give your body most of the energy it needs, help protect your muscles, and provide nutrients that aid digestion. Even if you're trying to lose weight, you shouldn't completely eliminate carbohydrates from your diet. The Glycemic Index Diet helps you choose foods that contain nutrients but will not cause spikes in your blood glucose levels.

As the following sections explain, different types of foods have different effects on blood glucose levels.

GOOD FATS

Fats are an important part of a healthy diet, providing essential fatty acids and delivering fat-soluble vitamins, and they are a great source of energizing fuel for your body. More important than just the amount of fat, it's the *types* of fat you eat that really matter. Saturated fats and trans fats, commonly termed "bad" fats, increase cholesterol and your risk of certain diseases, while "good" fats—monounsaturated fats, polyunsaturated fats, and omega-3s—protect your heart and support overall health. Here are some examples of foods with good fats:

Foods That Contain Good Fats

Almonds	Peanut butter
Avocados	Pecans
Cashews	Pistachios
Chia seeds	Salmon
Eggs	Sardines
Flaxseed	Sesame oil
Fish oil	Sesame seeds
Hazelnuts	Soymilk
Herring	Sunflower seeds
Macadamia nuts	Tofu
Mackerel	Trout
Olives	Tuna
Olive oil	Walnuts
Peanuts	

PROTEINS

Proteins (including legumes) have been shown to inhibit the rise in blood glucose. Eggs, fish, and nonfatty meat are very low on the glycemic index scale, too.

Low-GI

Almonds

Anchovies (canned)

Beans (dried or canned)

Canadian bacon

Chicken (skinless)

Cod

Eggs

Haddock

Lean beef

Lean ham (baked, boiled,
  or smoked)

Lentils

Mackerel (fresh or canned)

Low-fat cheese

Peanuts

Salmon (fresh, canned,
  or smoked)

Scallops

Shrimp

Tempeh

Tofu

Tuna (fresh or canned)

Turkey (skinless)

FOODS TO AVOID, FOODS TO ENJOY

The food tables in this book are intended to help you do your best to avoid foods with high glycemic index scores. As you've learned, the glycemic index scale ranks food from 0 to 100 based on how they affect your blood sugar levels. Carbohydrates are ranked according to how fast and how high they raised the blood sugar levels of individuals in clinical trials. Here is a quick overview of where some common foods lie on the glycemic index scale:

- *High (70 and higher):* white rice, brown rice, white bread, skinless baked white potato, baked red potato with skin, and watermelon
- *Medium (56 to 69):* sweet corn, bananas, pineapple, raisins, and certain types of ice cream
- *Low (55 and lower):* raw carrots, peanuts, raw apples, grapefruit, nonfat milk, kidney beans, and lentils

You can find the glycemic index scores of many foods on the Internet; the National Cancer Institute offers a downloadable file containing GI values on its website (http://appliedresearch.cancer.gov/tools/glycemic/). In Chapter 4, you'll find lists of many common foods and their glycemic loads.

TIPS FOR REDUCING BLOOD GLUCOSE LEVELS THROUGH DIET

Here are ten ways you can reduce your blood glucose levels by adjusting your diet.

1. Drink lots of water.

It is important to stay hydrated. If you normally drink soda or even diet soda, try drinking water instead. You can jazz up your water by substituting sparkling water for tap water, or by adding a lemon or lime slice.

2. Eat a high-protein diet.

Proteins help you feel fuller longer. In a study of teenage boys, those who ate a lot of protein as part of a low-GI diet stayed fuller longer and ate fewer calories. This fact did not change even when the boys increased their activity levels by exercising more.

3. Watch out for glucose in beverages.

Hidden glucose may be creeping into your diet via what you drink and how you drink it. There's a big difference in the amount of calories and the glycemic index score of black coffee versus a peppermint mocha with whipped cream. Other high-calorie indulgences include soda and juice. As you learned earlier, certain fruit juices have high glycemic index scores.

4. Plan menus in advance.

Planning your weekly menu in advance will go a long way toward helping you stay on course with eating low-GI foods. After you plan your menu, make a shopping list before going to the store.

5. Stick to your shopping list.

As stated above, it's a good idea to take a shopping list to the store. Then, once you're in the store, try to stick to the list. This will cut down on impulse purchases, which are usually items that aren't good for you and/or have high glycemic index scores.

6. Eat more veggies.

Almost all vegetables are low on the glycemic index scale. Filling up on vegetables is a great way to feel full and satisfied.

7. Watch your portion size.

Not all foods that have a low glycemic index score are low in fat or good for you. You must be aware of your serving size. Remembering to serve portions wisely is almost as important as the food choices you make. USDA food guide portion sizes include 1 slice of bread or ½ cup cooked cereal, rice, or pasta when consuming grains; 1 cup of raw leafy vegetables or ½ cup cooked vegetables; 1 medium fruit or ½ cup of cooked or canned fruit; 2 to 3 ounces of cooked lean meat, poultry, or fish; 6 to 12 nuts (depending on size) or 2 tablespoons of nut butter; and 1 cup of low-fat milk or yogurt or 1½ ounces reduced-fat cheese.

8. Be mindful of the state of your food.

Ripe fruit has more sugar in it than unripe fruit. Take bananas: if they're slightly green, they're hard and not very sweet, whereas ripe bananas are soft and sweet. The ripe banana is softer and sweeter because it has higher sugar content than the green banana. That doesn't mean you need to eat green bananas, though—just be aware that you may be taking in more sugar from a very ripe banana.

9. Find alternatives to satisfy sugar cravings.

If you crave sugar, there are some alternatives that have relatively low glycemic index scores. If you're craving ice cream, say, you could try low-fat frozen yogurt instead. Beware, though—some frozen yogurts are loaded with sugar. Try this: When you're *not* having a craving, go to your nearest health food store, look at the different flavors of frozen yogurt, and choose one you think you might like. That way, it's in your freezer waiting for you during your next craving. Or keep fresh fruit around and eat an apple or a bowl of berries when you're craving something sweet.

10. Choose foods that have low glycemic index scores.

Continue to use the glycemic index scale to choose carbohydrates and the other foods in your diet. Remember, you need to have carbs in your diet, but some food choices are better than others. For example, if you have a craving for pasta, a high-GI food, try whole-wheat pasta instead. Although whole wheat isn't low on the glycemic index scale, it doesn't cause the same spikes in your blood sugar as regular pasta.

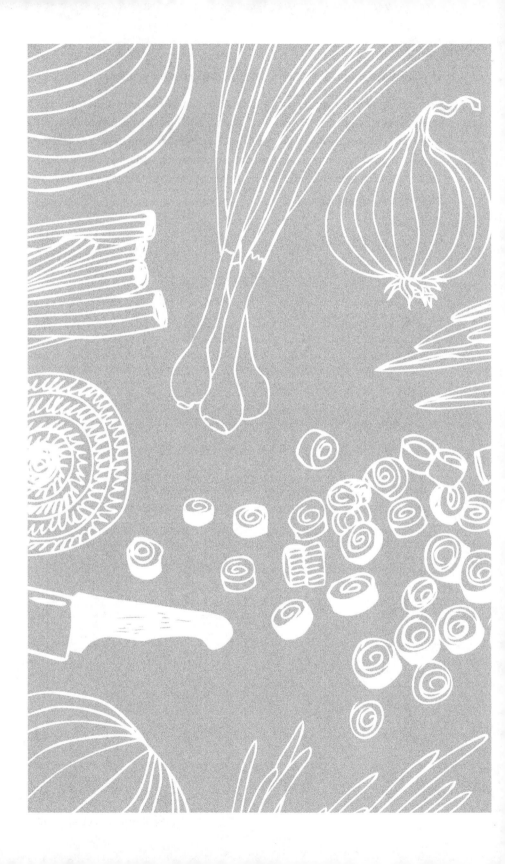

CHAPTER 3

Meal Planning with the Glycemic Index Diet

You've decided to take better control of your blood glucose levels and reduce the amount of sugar in your diet. Congratulations! Whatever your overall health goals, this is a wonderful step toward taking better care of yourself. It's always a good idea to write down what your commitments and goals are. And if you're diabetic, it's a good idea to take note of the range of blood sugar values that you want to maintain over the course of the day.

Give yourself a daily goal for your Glycemic Index Diet. For example, your goal might be to eat low-GI foods throughout the day or to maintain your blood sugar levels within a certain range. If your goal is to lose weight, your goal might be to eat less than the total amount of calories you've allotted yourself for the day. Every day that you meet your goal, give yourself a star for reaching that goal. When you've earned 14 stars, give yourself a small reward. Find a reward that's personal and doesn't involve eating. It might be to watch your favorite movie, to buy a book you've always wanted to read, or something else that's important to you. If you earn lots of stars over time (50 or more, say), give yourself a *big* reward.

Try to plan your meals for at least one week in advance. The 14-day menu offered here is a suggestion to help you get started. Feel free to substitute similar foods to suit your preferences; for instance, you can have a turkey sandwich instead of a roast beef sandwich, or a pear instead of an apple.

14-DAY MEAL PLAN

Week 1

SUNDAY

Breakfast
Scrambled eggs, bacon
Coffee (black or with light cream, no sugar), tea, water
Lunch
Salad* with baked chicken
Seltzer water
Dinner
Baked chicken, green beans, salad*
Snack
Frozen yogurt

MONDAY

Breakfast
Oatmeal with strawberries and pecans
Coffee, etc.
Lunch
Hummus with carrots and celery
Water or other low-calorie beverage
Dinner
Roast pork, broccoli, salad*
Snack
Apple

TUESDAY

Breakfast
Yogurt with fruit
Coffee, etc.
Lunch
Salad* with cheese

*Salads should include no more than 1 tablespoon of dressing.

Seltzer water

Dinner

Steak, spinach, salad*

Snack

Hummus with carrots and celery

WEDNESDAY

Breakfast

Oatmeal with mixed nuts

Coffee, etc.

Lunch

Quinoa salad

Water or other low-calorie beverage

Dinner

Salmon, spinach

Snack

Whole-wheat toast with peanut butter

THURSDAY

Breakfast

Yogurt with mixed nuts

Coffee, etc.

Lunch

Salad* with baked chicken

Seltzer water

Dinner

Whole-wheat pasta with tomato sauce

Snack

Yogurt

FRIDAY

Breakfast

Oatmeal with strawberries and pecans

Coffee, etc.

Lunch
Roast beef sandwich on whole-wheat bread
Water or other low-calorie beverage
Dinner
Baked chicken, green beans, salad*
Snack
A bowl of mixed berries

SATURDAY

Breakfast
Fruit salad, boiled egg
Coffee, etc.
Lunch
Tomato soup, salad*
Seltzer water
Dinner
Salmon, mushrooms, broccoli
Snack
Frozen yogurt

Week 2

SUNDAY

Breakfast
Yogurt with fruit
Coffee, etc.
Lunch
Roast beef sandwich on whole-wheat bread, side salad of cucumbers
and tomatoes
Seltzer water
Dinner
Whole-wheat pasta with tomato sauce, salad
Snack
Frozen yogurt

MONDAY

Breakfast
Fruit salad, boiled egg
Coffee, etc.
Lunch
Salad* with baked chicken
Seltzer water
Dinner
Steak, spinach, salad*
Snack
Apple

TUESDAY

Breakfast
Oatmeal with mixed nuts
Coffee, etc.
Lunch
Tomato soup, salad*
Water or other low-calorie beverage
Dinner
Roast pork, broccoli, salad*
Snack
Hummus with carrots and celery

WEDNESDAY

Breakfast
Yogurt with mixed nuts
Coffee, etc.
Lunch
Hummus with carrots and celery
Tea
Dinner
Tofu stir-fry with vegetables
Snack
Whole-wheat toast with peanut butter

THURSDAY

Breakfast
Oatmeal with strawberries and pecans
Coffee, etc.
Lunch
Salad* with cheese
Seltzer water
Dinner
Steak, spinach, salad*
Snack
Yogurt

FRIDAY

Breakfast
Yogurt with fruit
Coffee, etc.
Lunch
Quinoa salad
Tea
Dinner
Halibut, brown rice, peas
Snack
A bowl of mixed berries

SATURDAY

Breakfast
Scrambled eggs, bacon
Coffee, etc.
Lunch
Salad* with baked chicken
Seltzer water
Dinner
Baked chicken, green beans, salad*
Snack
Frozen yogurt

SHOPPING TIPS

The key to successfully following a meal plan is preparation. Before you shop, plan out your meal and snack menu for the week. Make a list of items that you intend to buy and stick to the items on your list. When you go shopping, try to stay focused on your list and not be distracted by other, less healthy items. It's a good idea to go shopping right after you eat a full meal. This will cut down on cravings, which can lead to impulse buying. Try to avoid making last-minute buying decisions, as these tend to result in less-healthy food choices. Reread the tips on page 27 for reducing blood glucose levels through diet to get into the right frame of mind before you head to the grocery store.

DINING OUT

Dining out can be the most difficult time to stick to an eating regimen. Reading through the tables in Chapter 4 of this book will help you know which types of foods have low glycemic loads. Here are a few other ideas that can help when you eat out:

Try to plan ahead: If you're going out with a group of friends, suggest restaurants or styles of cuisine that are more likely to have healthy food choices. For example, Italian cuisine features a number of high-GI foods, such as pasta, so that might not be your best choice. Once a restaurant is agreed on, you can likely find their menu on their website. That way, you can check the glycemic index scores of certain foods and make your choices ahead of time to avoid making impulsive decisions.

Avoid fried foods: Since they have higher fat content, fried foods like french fries actually have a lower GI score than their natural counterparts, like potatoes. But even with a relatively lower score, fried foods are still too high-GI to be healthy.

Avoid foods with lots of sauces: Sauces make foods taste good, but they are often a hidden source of extra sugar and carbohydrates.

Skip the white rice and white noodles: These foods are among the highest-scoring items on the glycemic index scale. Happily, some Asian cuisines have tasty dishes that are low on the glycemic index scale. But make sure you skip the white rice (or white noodles) to keep the GI score of your meal low.

Substitute whole grains for pastas and breads: If you're at an Italian restaurant and don't have a variety of choices, ask your waiter if they offer a whole-wheat substitute for the pasta in your dish. (This option is becoming more common.) Also, try to avoid any free bread that's placed on your table—you can ask the waiter to simply take it away if your dining companions agree. If you have to eat some bread, make it whole wheat.

CHAPTER 4

Glycemic Load Tables

The glycemic index scale measures how quickly foods break down into sugar in your bloodstream. High-glycemic foods turn into blood sugar quickly. While a food's glycemic index is important and can help you choose which foods to eat, the GI value doesn't tell you how many carbohydrates you're getting per serving. That's where a food's glycemic load number comes in handy. The glycemic load is calculated by taking the amount of carbohydrates in each serving, multiplying that figure by the food's glycemic index score, and then dividing that number by 100.

Consuming 1 glycemic load unit is effectively the same as consuming 1 gram of glucose. As a rule of thumb, glycemic loads above 20 are considered high and glycemic loads below 10 are considered low. Your goal should be to choose foods with a low glycemic load whenever possible. The serving sizes in these tables have been rounded to whole numbers for convenience.

Breads		
	Serving Size (in grams)	Glycemic Load (grams/serving)
Bagel (plain)	89	33
Baguette	30	15
Cornbread	60	30
Corn tortilla	24	7
Croissant	57	17
French bread	64	30
Gluten-free white bread	30	10
Hamburger bun	30	9
Kaiser roll	30	12
Oat-bran bread	30	9
Pumpernickel bread	30	7
Pita bread (white)	30	10

Breads		
	Serving Size (in grams)	Glycemic Load (grams/serving)
Pizza crust	99	43
White bread	30	10
Whole-wheat bread	28	7
Whole-wheat tortilla	50	8

Beverages		
	Serving Size (in milliliters)*	Glycemic Load (grams/serving)
Apple juice (unsweetened)	250	30
Carrot juice	235	43
Cola	250	26
Cranberry juice cocktail	250	24
Gatorade	250	15
Grapefruit juice (unsweetened)	250	11
Hot chocolate (made from a mix with hot water)	250	11
Orange juice	250	26
Orange soda	250	23
Raspberry smoothie	250	33
Soymilk	235	4
Tomato juice	250	9
Alcohol		
Beer	355	<15
Red wine	175	<15
White wine	175	<15

Note: 250 milliliters equals approximately 8.5 ounces.

Fruits

	Serving Size (in grams)	Glycemic Load (grams/serving)
Apple	120	6
Apricot	120	5
Banana (ripe)	120	16
Cantaloupe	120	4
Cherries	120	3
Dates	60	42
Figs	60	16
Grapefruit	120	3
Grapes	120	11
Kiwi	120	5
Mango	120	8
Orange	120	5
Papaya	140	6
Peach	120	4
Pear	120	4
Pineapple	155	12
Plum	66	2
Raisins	60	28
Strawberries	120	1
Watermelon	120	4

Proteins

	Serving Size (in grams unless otherwise noted)	Glycemic Load (grams/serving)
Almonds	95	0
Baked beans	150	6
Black beans	150	7
Black-eyed peas	150	10
Cashews	50	3
Chickpeas	150	3

Proteins

	Serving Size (in grams unless otherwise noted)	Glycemic Load (grams/serving)
Eggs	2 large	0
Kidney beans	150	6
Lentils	150	5
Lima beans	241	7
Navy beans	150	9
Peanuts	50	0
Pecans	109	0
Pinto beans	171	12
Salmon	178	0
Soybeans	150	1
Meat		
Beef (steak)	10 oz.	<15
Chicken	1 breast	<15
Lamb	3-4 oz.	<15
Pork	2-5 oz.	<15

Cereals and Grains

	Serving Size (in grams)	Glycemic Load (grams/serving)
Basmati rice	150	28
Brown rice	150	16
Buckwheat	150	16
Bulgur	150	12
Cream of Wheat	250	17
Cornflakes	30	23
Couscous	150	9
Millet	150	25
Muesli	30	16
Oatmeal	250	13

Cereals and Grains

	Serving Size (in grams)	Glycemic Load (grams/serving)
Pearled barley	150	12
Puffed wheat	30	17
Quinoa	150	13
Raisin bran	30	12
White rice	150	43
Wild rice	150	18

Vegetables

	Serving Size (in grams)	Glycemic Load (grams/serving)
Artichoke	80	0
Beets (canned)	246	10
Beets (fresh)	80	5
Broccoli	78	0
Cabbage	75	0
Carrots	80	3
Cauliflower	100	0
Celery	110	1
Collard greens	190	4
Corn	166	61
Cucumber	80	0
Green beans	110	3
Mushrooms	70	0
Parsnips	213	36
Peas	150	3
Rutabaga	150	7
Spinach	30	0
Sweet potato	150	17
Tomato	123	2
White potato	150	33

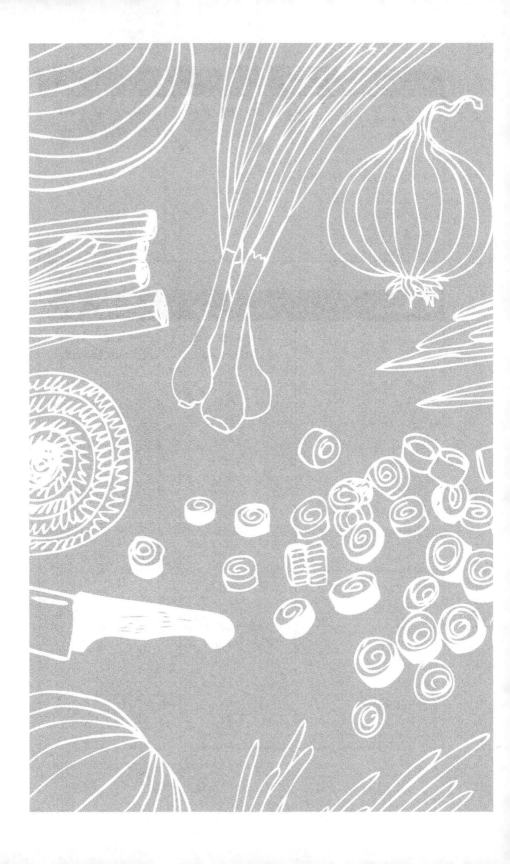

PART TWO

Recipes

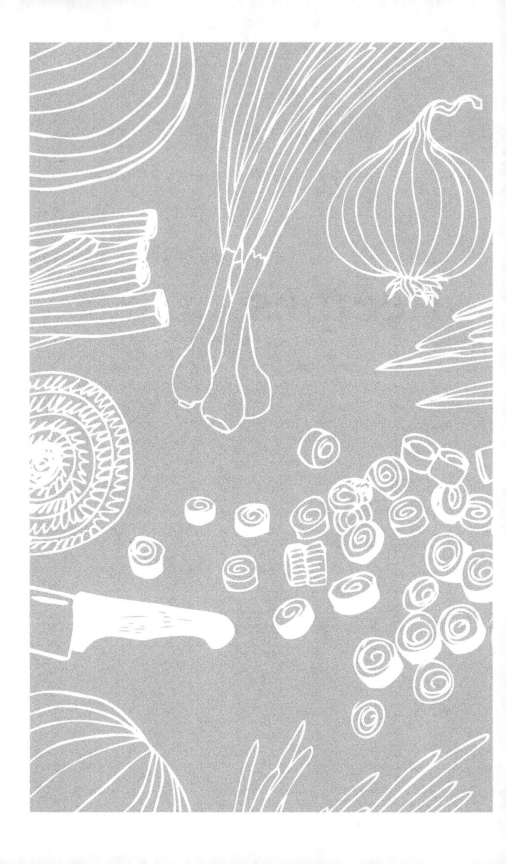

CHAPTER 5

Breakfast

Apple-Kale Wake-Up Smoothie

SERVES 1

A bit tangy, a bit sweet, and full of the refreshing flavor of greens, this powerful smoothie will make you feel ready to start your day. If you're in a hurry, whip up a quick batch, pour it into an insulated travel cup, and enjoy it on your morning commute.

¾ CUP STEMMED, COARSELY CHOPPED KALE LEAVES

1 APPLE, PEELED, CORED, AND COARSELY CHOPPED

½ CUP COLD UNSWEETENED ALMOND MILK

½ CUP COLD UNSWEETENED APPLE JUICE

1 TABLESPOON FRESHLY SQUEEZED LEMON JUICE

Place all of the ingredients in a blender and process until smooth. Serve immediately.

Very Berry Breakfast Smoothie

SERVES 1

This bright, sweet smoothie will help keep you healthy with a hearty dose of antioxidants, plus healthy fat, a bit of protein, and other essential nutrients, including iron, magnesium, phosphorus, zinc, copper, and manganese.

1 CUP COLD UNSWEETENED COCONUT MILK

⅔ CUP FROZEN BERRIES (BLUEBERRIES, BLACKBERRIES, STRAWBERRIES, RASPBERRIES, OR A MIXTURE)

⅓ CUP CASHEWS

1 TEASPOON PURE VANILLA EXTRACT

1 TEASPOON HONEY

Place all of the ingredients in a blender and process until smooth. Serve immediately.

Tropical Yogurt Parfait

SERVES 4

Parfaits make for quick and healthy breakfasts with infinite variations. Use seasonal fruits and mix things up by adding nuts or toasted whole-grain cereals for a bit of crunch. Use clear glasses to show off the colorful layers and serve with long-handled spoons. You can even make these in mason jars and store, covered, in the fridge for a week's worth of workday breakfasts.

4 CUPS PLAIN LOW-FAT GREEK YOGURT
1 CUP DICED PINEAPPLE, FRESH OR CANNED, DRAINED
1 MANGO, PEELED AND DICED
¼ CUP UNSWEETENED COCONUT FLAKES, TOASTED

1. Line up 4 bowls, cups, or tall glasses and fill the bottom of each one with a large dollop of yogurt. Add a layer of pineapple and mango to each glass, and then a layer of coconut. Add another layer of yogurt, then another layer each of pineapple and mango.

2. Top with a final layer of yogurt and sprinkle with the remaining coconut.

Pumpkin-Spice Steel-Cut Oatmeal

SERVES 2

Steel-cut oats differ from old-fashioned rolled oats in that, instead of being rolled into flat flakes, the whole toasted oat grain is simply cut into chunks. When cooked, steel-cut oats maintain a chewier texture, but nutritionally, the two types are nearly identical.

Whichever type of oats you choose, eating oatmeal will help you ward off cardio-vascular disease, diabetes, hypertension, and obesity. This hearty recipe tastes like pumpkin pie in a bowl, perfect for a chilly fall morning. You can add berries or diced pears, if you like, for a bit of added sweetness.

1½ CUPS WATER

½ CUP STEEL-CUT OATS

PINCH OF SALT

¼ CUP CANNED PUMPKIN PUREE

¼ CUP UNSWEETENED APPLESAUCE

⅛ TEASPOON GROUND CINNAMON

PINCH OF GROUND CLOVES

PINCH OF GROUND NUTMEG

1 TO 2 TABLESPOONS WHOLE MILK (OPTIONAL)

2 TABLESPOONS CHOPPED TOASTED WALNUTS OR PECANS (OPTIONAL)

1. In a medium saucepan, bring the water to a boil. Stir in the oats and salt, and then reduce the heat to low. Simmer, uncovered, stirring occasionally, until the oats are tender, 20 to 25 minutes.

2. Stir in the pumpkin, applesauce, cinnamon, cloves, and nutmeg and cook, stirring, for another 5 minutes.

3. Transfer the oatmeal to a serving bowl, stir in the milk, and sprinkle the nuts on top, if using. Serve hot.

Vanilla-Blueberry Bulgur Cereal

SERVES 2

Bulgur is more commonly seen in savory dishes, but since it's easy to cook and loaded with fiber, it makes a great hot breakfast cereal as well. Sweetened with antioxidant-rich blueberries, this healthy cereal will warm you up on a chilly morning.

1 CUP WATER

½ CUP MEDIUM-GRAIN BULGUR

PINCH OF SALT

¼ CUP MILK

1 TEASPOON PURE VANILLA EXTRACT

1 CUP FRESH OR FROZEN BLUEBERRIES

1. In a medium saucepan, combine the water, bulgur, and salt and bring to a boil.

2. Immediately cover the pot, remove it from heat, and let stand until the water is fully absorbed, about 10 minutes.

3. Stir in the milk, vanilla, and blueberries and serve hot.

Flax and Almond Butter Hot Cereal

SERVES 1

This high-fiber, high-protein cereal will wake you up and keep you going all the way until lunch. Feel free to substitute almond milk, coconut milk, or soymilk for the dairy milk, if desired.

¼ CUP FLAXSEED MEAL
½ CUP BOILING WATER
2 TABLESPOONS MILK
2 TABLESPOONS ALMOND BUTTER
2 TEASPOONS HONEY
¼ TEASPOON GROUND CINNAMON

1. Place the flaxseed meal in a bowl and pour the boiling water over it. Stir to mix.

2. Add the milk, almond butter, honey, and cinnamon and let sit until it thickened, 2 minutes or so. Serve immediately.

Blueberry Granola Bars

MAKES 12 BARS

These protein- and fiber-packed bars are great to have around for those mornings when you have to eat breakfast on the run. They also make great snacks.

COOKING SPRAY

1⅓ CUPS WHOLE-WHEAT FLOUR

¼ CUP WHEAT BRAN

2 TEASPOONS BAKING POWDER

1 TEASPOON GROUND CINNAMON

1 TEASPOON GROUND ALLSPICE

½ TEASPOON GROUND GINGER

½ TEASPOON SALT

1½ CUPS ROLLED OATS

1 CUP DRIED BLUEBERRIES

¼ CUP SUNFLOWER SEEDS

¼ CUP SESAME SEEDS

2 TABLESPOONS FLAXSEED

¾ CUP UNSWEETENED APPLESAUCE

½ CUP UNSWEETENED APPLE JUICE

⅓ CUP HONEY

3 LARGE EGGS, LIGHTLY BEATEN

2 TEASPOONS VEGETABLE OIL

1. Preheat the oven to 400°F and spray a 9-by-13-inch baking dish with cooking spray.

2. In a large mixing bowl, stir together the flour, bran, baking powder, cinnamon, allspice, ginger, and salt. Add the oats, blueberries, sunflower seeds, sesame seeds, and flaxseed and stir to combine. Add the applesauce, apple juice, honey, eggs, and oil, and stir to mix well.

3. Pour the mixture into the prepared baking dish and use a spatula to even out and smooth the top. Bake until lightly browned, 18 to 20 minutes. Place the pan on a wire rack to cool to room temperature. Cut into 12 bars and serve. Store the bars in an airtight container at room temperature for up to a week.

Apple-Cinnamon Pancakes

SERVES 4

These whole-grain pancakes get their fiber from both whole-wheat flour and oats. Sweetened with shredded apples, they don't even need any syrup or other sweetener. The addition of cinnamon makes them taste just like Mom's apple pie. Serve them with unsweetened applesauce or yogurt on the side, if desired.

¾ CUP WHOLE WHEAT FLOUR

½ CUP OLD-FASHIONED ROLLED OATS

1 TEASPOON BAKING POWDER

½ TEASPOON GROUND CINNAMON

2 LARGE EGGS

¾ CUP 1 PERCENT MILK, PLUS MORE IF NEEDED

1 TEASPOON PURE VANILLA EXTRACT

1 CUP PEELED, SHREDDED APPLE

2 TABLESPOONS BUTTER, MELTED

1. In a large bowl, combine the flour, oats, baking powder, and cinnamon.

2. In a medium bowl, whisk together the eggs, milk, and vanilla. Stir the egg mixture into the dry mixture and then stir in the shredded apple. If the mixture seems thick, add a bit more milk.

3. Heat a large skillet over medium-high heat and brush with a bit of the melted butter. Drop the batter by the ¼ cupful into the pan, leaving space for the pancakes to spread. Cook until bubbles form on the tops and the bottoms are golden brown, 2 to 3 minutes. Flip the pancakes and cook until golden brown on the second side, another 2 to 3 minutes. Repeat with the remaining batter, brushing the skillet with butter between each batch.

4. Serve hot.

Banana-Nut Bread

SERVES 8

Choose the ripest bananas you can find to infuse this moist banana bread with intense banana flavor. It gets lots of protein from the almond flour, eggs, and walnuts, and plenty of fiber from the buckwheat flour. Serve it alongside a bowl of fresh fruit.

COOKING SPRAY

1½ CUPS BUCKWHEAT FLOUR

½ CUP ALMOND FLOUR

½ CUP WALNUTS, TOASTED AND CHOPPED

2 TEASPOONS BAKING POWDER

2 LARGE RIPE BANANAS, PEELED

2 LARGE EGGS, BEATEN

½ CUP HONEY

½ CUP COCONUT OIL

1 TEASPOON GROUND CINNAMON

1. Preheat the oven to 350°F and spray a 4-by-8-inch loaf pan with cooking spray.

2. In a medium bowl, combine the buckwheat flour, almond flour, walnuts, and baking powder.

3. In a large bowl, mash the bananas. Whisk in the eggs, honey, coconut oil, and cinnamon. Add the dry ingredients and stir to mix well.

4. Transfer the batter to the prepared loaf pan and bake for 50 minutes. Cool in the pan on a rack for about 20 minutes. Remove from the pan and slice. Wrap any leftovers in plastic and store in the refrigerator for up to 4 days.

Baked Eggs with Mushrooms, Tomatoes, and Greens

SERVES 4

This simple egg breakfast is easy to make, looks gorgeous, and is loaded with vegetables.

COOKING SPRAY
12 CHERRY TOMATOES, HALVED
8 CREMINI OR BUTTON MUSHROOMS, SLICED
1 GARLIC CLOVE, THINLY SLICED
2 TEASPOONS OLIVE OIL
½ TEASPOON SALT
8 OUNCES BABY SPINACH
4 LARGE EGGS
2 TABLESPOONS GRATED PARMESAN CHEESE
1 TABLESPOON MINCED FRESH PARSLEY

1. Preheat the oven to 400°F and spray four 8-ounce ramekins with cooking spray.

2. Divide the tomatoes, mushrooms, and garlic evenly among the prepared ramekins. Drizzle the oil over the top and sprinkle with the salt. Bake for 10 minutes.

3. While the ramekins are in the oven, wilt the spinach by placing it in a colander and pouring boiling water over it. Drain well and squeeze out as much water as you can.

4. Remove the ramekins from the oven and add the spinach to the ramekins, dividing evenly.

5. Make a well in the middle of each ramekin and crack 1 egg into each. Bake until the egg whites are set but the yolks are still a bit runny, 8 to 10 minutes. Sprinkle the Parmesan cheese and parsley over the tops and serve.

Spring Pea and Mint Frittata with Goat Cheese and Pancetta

SERVES 6

This pretty frittata is quick to make and can be served hot, warm, or at room temperature, so it's a great make-ahead brunch dish or an everyday breakfast dish. Store leftover wedges in the fridge and reheat in the microwave for a fast weekday morning breakfast. (If you can't find pancetta, substitute thick-cut bacon.)

2 TEASPOONS OLIVE OIL

1 SMALL SHALLOT, DICED

1 GARLIC CLOVE, MINCED

2 OUNCES PANCETTA, DICED

2 CUPS FROZEN PEAS

8 LARGE EGGS

2 TABLESPOONS MILK

¾ TEASPOON SALT

4 OUNCES GOAT CHEESE, CRUMBLED

2 TABLESPOONS CHOPPED FRESH MINT

1. Preheat the oven to 450°F.

2. In a large, oven-safe nonstick skillet, heat the oil over medium-high heat. Add the shallot, garlic, and pancetta and cook, stirring frequently, until the shallot is soft, about 5 minutes. Add the peas and cook just until they thaw, 1 to 2 minutes.

3. Meanwhile, in a medium bowl, whisk together the eggs, milk, and salt. Add half of the goat cheese to the eggs along with the mint and whisk to combine. Pour the egg mixture over the vegetables in the skillet.

4. Transfer the skillet to the oven and cook until the top is almost set, 8 to 10 minutes. Turn on the broiler.

5. Crumble the remaining goat cheese over the top and transfer the skillet to the broiler. Broil until the cheese is golden brown and bubbling, 2 to 3 minutes. Cut into wedges and serve.

Zucchini and Egg Breakfast Muffins

MAKES 24 MINI MUFFINS

These quick little frittata bites make a fantastic grab-and-go breakfast, but they're so adorable that they also make for perfect party food. And they're full of fresh vegetables and protein, too.

COOKING SPRAY
1 TABLESPOON OLIVE OIL
2 SHALLOTS, MINCED
2 GARLIC CLOVES, MINCED
2 SMALL ZUCCHINI, GRATED
2 TABLESPOONS MINCED FRESH BASIL
3 TABLESPOONS WHOLE-WHEAT FLOUR
2¼ CUPS WHOLE MILK, DIVIDED
4 LARGE EGGS, LIGHTLY BEATEN
¾ TEASPOON KOSHER SALT
⅛ TEASPOON GROUND NUTMEG
¼ CUP GRATED GRUYÈRE OR PARMESAN CHEESE

1. Preheat the oven to 450°F and spray a nonstick mini muffin tin with cooking spray.

2. In a large nonstick skillet, heat the oil over medium-high heat. Add the shallots and garlic and cook, stirring, until the shallot begins to soften, about 3 minutes. Add the zucchini and cook, stirring, until the zucchini is softened, about 4 minutes. Remove from the heat and stir in the basil.

3. In a medium bowl, whisk together the flour and ½ cup of the milk. Add the eggs and the remaining 1¾ cups milk and whisk to combine. Whisk in the salt and nutmeg.

continued ▶

4. Divide the cheese evenly among the muffin cups. Next, place a spoonful of the zucchini mixture into each muffin cup. Pour the egg mixture over the top of the vegetables.

5. Bake until puffed and golden, 16 to 18 minutes. Remove from the oven and let cool for 10 minutes or so before carefully removing each muffin. Serve immediately or cool to room temperature on a rack.

6. Store the muffins in a covered container in the refrigerator for up to 3 days, or freeze in a single layer and then transfer to a zipper-top plastic bag and keep frozen for up to 3 months. Reheat the frozen muffins on a baking sheet in a 400°F oven for about 10 minutes.

The Creamiest Scrambled Eggs

SERVES 4

In this custard-like dish, eggs are cooked slowly over boiling water, making them super creamy. A splash of vinegar in the eggs keeps them tender. It's one of those rare dishes that shines as much for its deliciousness as for its simplicity.

8 LARGE EGGS

¼ CUP 1 PERCENT MILK

1 TABLESPOON WHITE VINEGAR

¾ TEASPOON SALT

1 TABLESPOON MINCED FRESH HERBS (BASIL, OREGANO, THYME, PARSLEY,
    SAGE, OR A COMBINATION), PLUS ADDITIONAL FOR GARNISH

1 TABLESPOON UNSALTED BUTTER

GROUND BLACK PEPPER

1. Bring water to a boil in the bottom of a double boiler over medium-high heat. Reduce the heat to maintain a simmer.

2. In a large bowl, whisk together the eggs, milk, vinegar, and salt. Whisk in the 1 tablespoon fresh herbs.

3. In the top half of the double boiler, melt the butter, and then add the egg mixture. Cook gently, stirring frequently, until the egg mixture is just set but not dry, 15 to 20 minutes. Serve immediately, seasoned with pepper and garnished with the remaining herbs.

Crispy Quinoa Cakes with Poached Eggs and Pesto

SERVES 4

These crispy, golden quinoa cakes are a great substitute for English muffins or other bread as a base for poached eggs. They're full of flavor and loaded with protein, fiber, and other nutrients. Serve alongside sautéed spinach, Swiss chard, or kale, if desired.

1½ CUPS COOKED QUINOA

1 LARGE EGG, LIGHTLY BEATEN

2 TABLESPOONS MINCED ONION

1 SMALL GARLIC CLOVE, MINCED

¼ CUP WHOLE-WHEAT FLOUR

¼ CUP GRATED PARMESAN CHEESE

¾ TEASPOON SALT

¼ TEASPOON GROUND BLACK PEPPER

OIL FOR FRYING

4 LARGE EGGS

¼ CUP PESTO

PARMESAN CHEESE

1. Fill a large saucepan with water and bring to a boil over high heat.

2. In a medium bowl, combine the quinoa, egg, onion, garlic, flour, cheese, salt, and pepper and mix well. Form the mixture into 4 large or 8 small patties.

3. In a large skillet, heat the oil over medium-high heat. Add the quinoa patties, in batches if necessary to avoid crowding, and cook until golden brown, about 3 minutes per side. Transfer the cooked patties to a paper towel–lined plate to drain. When all of the patties have been cooked, place them on serving plates.

4. Meanwhile, reduce the heat under the pot of water to low so that the water is just simmering. Carefully crack the eggs into the water and cook for 4 minutes. Use a slotted spoon to remove the eggs from the water and place one on each plate, on top of the quinoa patties. Top with a dollop of pesto and grate Parmesan cheese over the top. Serve immediately.

Chorizo and Egg Breakfast Burritos

SERVES 4

Make this spicy egg burrito with either chorizo or a soy-based substitute. Either way, the intense spices will add plenty of flavor, while the veggies and whole-wheat tortillas pack in nutrients and fiber.

4 LARGE WHOLE-WHEAT TORTILLAS

2 TEASPOONS OLIVE OR CANOLA OIL

6 OUNCES MEXICAN-STYLE CHORIZO OR SOY CHORIZO

½ SMALL ONION, DICED

1 RED BELL PEPPER, SEEDED AND DICED

8 OUNCES BABY SPINACH

8 LARGE EGGS

2 TABLESPOONS MILK

1 TEASPOON SALT

½ TEASPOON GROUND BLACK PEPPER

½ CUP SHREDDED SHARP CHEDDAR CHEESE

COOKING SPRAY

¼ CUP SALSA

1 SMALL AVOCADO, CUBED

1. Preheat the oven to 400°F and wrap the tortillas in aluminum foil. Place the tortillas in the oven to warm.

2. In a large nonstick skillet, heat the oil over medium-high heat. Add the chorizo, onion, and bell pepper and cook, stirring and breaking up the sausage with a wooden spoon, until the onion and pepper are softened and slightly browned, about 8 minutes. Stir in the spinach and continue to cook until it is just wilted. Transfer the mixture to a medium bowl.

continued ▶

3. In a large bowl, whisk together the eggs, milk, salt, and black pepper. Add the cheese and stir to mix. Wipe the skillet out with a paper towel, spray it with cooking spray, and reheat it over medium-high heat. Reduce the heat to low and add the egg mixture. Cook, stirring frequently with a spatula, until the eggs are fully cooked but not dry.

4. Remove the tortillas from the oven and fill each with equal amounts of the eggs and the sausage mixture.

5. Top with salsa and avocado, roll up, and serve.

CHAPTER 6

Snacks and Appetizers

Curry-Lime Almonds

SERVES 8

Almonds are a great source of heart-healthy monounsaturated fats—the kind found in olive oil—as well as vitamins and minerals like vitamin E, magnesium, and potassium. Here they make a spicy snack that's full of protein and low in carbohydrates.

2 TABLESPOONS FRESHLY SQUEEZED LIME JUICE

2 TABLESPOONS CURRY POWDER

½ TEASPOON SALT

¼ TEASPOON CAYENNE (OPTIONAL)

2 CUPS BLANCHED ALMONDS

1. Preheat the oven to 250°F.

2. In a medium bowl, whisk together the lime juice, curry powder, salt, and cayenne (if using) until well combined. Add the almonds and stir to coat. Spread in an even layer on a large baking sheet.

3. Bake, stirring occasionally, until beginning to brown, 45 to 50 minutes. Cool completely and then serve, or store in an airtight container at room temperature for up to 1 week.

Crispy Parmesan Kale Chips

SERVES 4

These crispy, crunchy, salty, cheesy chips are a fantastic healthy alternative to potato chips or any other salty snack you might be craving. Kale is extremely low in calories and is one of the most nutrient-dense foods on the planet.

1 LARGE BUNCH CURLY-LEAF KALE

2 TABLESPOONS OLIVE OIL

¼ CUP GRATED PARMESAN CHEESE

SALT TO TASTE

1. Preheat the oven to 375°F.

2. Make sure the kale is very dry. Tear the kale into bite-sized pieces and toss in a large bowl with the olive oil.

3. Lay the kale in a single layer on a large baking sheet, sprinkle with the Parmesan and a pinch or two of salt, and bake in the preheated oven until crispy, 10 to 15 minutes. Serve immediately or store in an airtight container at room temperature for up to 3 days.

Creamy Garlic Hummus

SERVES 6

Homemade hummus has the bright flavors of fresh garlic, lemon, and herbs that just can't be duplicated by store-bought versions. This quick hummus is extra creamy thanks to the addition of Greek yogurt. As a bonus, the yogurt also substitutes for some of the oil and tahini found in traditional hummus, making it lower in fat, too. Serve this tasty dip with a platter of raw veggies for a healthy snack or appetizer.

½ CUP FRESH PARSLEY LEAVES

2 GARLIC CLOVES

1 (15-OUNCE) CAN CHICKPEAS, RINSED AND DRAINED

½ CUP PLAIN LOW-FAT GREEK YOGURT

2 TABLESPOONS TAHINI (SESAME PASTE)

2 TABLESPOONS FRESHLY SQUEEZED LEMON JUICE

1 TABLESPOON OLIVE OIL

1. Process the parsley and garlic in a food processor to mince well.

2. Add the chickpeas to the food processor and process until smooth.

3. Add the yogurt, tahini, lemon juice, and olive oil and process to blend well. If the mixture is too thick, add water, 1 tablespoon at a time, until you achieve the desired consistency. Serve immediately, garnished with additional parsley, or cover and refrigerate for up to 3 days.

Warm Citrus Olives with Almonds

This is a great way to dress up a bowl of olives or nuts for a party. They are best made just before serving, but if you want to make them ahead, simply leave out the almonds and then add them when you heat the olives up before serving.

2 TABLESPOONS OLIVE OIL

ZEST OF 1 LEMON OR SMALL ORANGE

½ TEASPOON SMOKED PAPRIKA

¼ TEASPOON CRUSHED RED PEPPER FLAKES

1 CUP CURED BLACK OLIVES, SUCH AS KALAMATA

2 CUPS UNSALTED ALMONDS, TOASTED

1. In a medium saucepan, heat the olive oil over medium heat. Reduce the heat to low and add the citrus zest, paprika, and red pepper flakes. Cook until the mixture becomes fragrant, 2 to 3 minutes.

2. Stir in the olives and almonds and cook, stirring, until they are warmed through, 2 to 3 minutes.

3. Let sit in the pan for 10 minutes or so to let the flavors meld, then transfer the mixture to a serving bowl using a slotted spoon (discard the excess oil). Serve warm with a small bowl for discarded olive pits.

Roasted Cauliflower with Tahini Dip

SERVES 6

Roasted vegetables are always crowd-pleasers. Here, healthy cauliflower is roasted to a golden brown and served alongside a nutty and tangy tahini dip. Tahini paste, made from sesame seeds, is full of good-for-your-bones calcium.

CAULIFLOWER:

OLIVE OIL COOKING SPRAY

1 HEAD CAULIFLOWER

2 TEASPOONS GROUND CUMIN

½ TEASPOON SALT

½ TEASPOON GROUND BLACK PEPPER

TAHINI DIP:

½ CUP PLAIN LOW-FAT YOGURT

½ CUP FRESHLY SQUEEZED LEMON JUICE

¼ CUP TAHINI

1 GARLIC CLOVE, MINCED

¾ TEASPOON SALT

¼ TEASPOON GROUND BLACK PEPPER

1. Preheat the oven to 400°F and spray a large nonstick baking sheet with olive oil spray.

2. Slice the cauliflower into 1-inch-thick slices or separate into small florets. Arrange the pieces on the prepared baking sheet. Spray the cauliflower with additional olive oil spray and then sprinkle the cumin, salt, and pepper evenly over the top. Roast for 10 minutes, then turn the cauliflower pieces over and continue to roast until golden brown, about 10 minutes more. Transfer the cauliflower to a serving platter.

3. In a small bowl, combine the yogurt, lemon juice, tahini, garlic, salt, and pepper and stir to mix well. Place the dip in a decorative serving bowl on the platter alongside the roasted cauliflower and serve.

Deviled Eggs with Bacon and Chives

SERVES 8

Deviled eggs are quite versatile. They're perfect to bring to a potluck or to serve at a cocktail party. These days, you even see them on the appetizer menus of ChiChi's restaurants. This version includes bits of crispy, smoky bacon for extra flavor.

12 HARD-BOILED LARGE EGGS
¼ CUP MAYONNAISE
1 TEASPOON UNSEASONED RICE VINEGAR
¼ TEASPOON SALT
¼ TEASPOON GROUND BLACK PEPPER
10 SLICES BACON, COOKED AND MINCED
2 TABLESPOONS MINCED FRESH CHIVES
PINCH OF SWEET OR SMOKED PAPRIKA

1. Carefully peel the eggs and slice them in half lengthwise. Remove the yolks and put them in a medium bowl. Arrange the whites face-up on a serving platter.

2. Mash the yolks and then add the mayonnaise, vinegar, salt, and pepper. Mix with a fork until well combined. Add the bacon and chives and stir to mix in thoroughly.

3. Pipe or spoon the yolk mixture into the whites. Sprinkle with the paprika and serve.

Crispy Prosciutto Cups with Peaches, Arugula, and Basil

MAKES 24

This simple recipe transforms a few simple but delicious ingredients into an impressive appetizer. Crisp prosciutto makes an ideal basket for peppery greens and sweet peaches.

12 THIN SLICES PROSCIUTTO, HALVED CROSSWISE

4 CUPS LIGHTLY PACKED ARUGULA, TRIMMED

2 TEASPOONS OLIVE OIL

¼ TEASPOON GROUND BLACK PEPPER

4 PEACHES, PEELED AND DICED

12 LARGE BASIL LEAVES, CUT INTO THIN RIBBONS

1. Preheat the oven to 375°F.

2. Press 1 piece of prosciutto into each cup of a mini muffin tin, arranging it so that it makes a cup. Bake until crisp, 12 to 15 minutes. Gently transfer the prosciutto cups to a wire rack to cool.

3. In a large bowl, gently toss the arugula with the olive oil and pepper.

4. Arrange the prosciutto cups on a serving platter. Place several arugula leaves in each cup. Top with a spoonful of the diced peaches and a few ribbons of basil. Serve immediately.

Thai Basil-Mint Chicken in Lettuce Leaves

SERVES 8

Crackers and chips are the fallback vehicles for getting delicious morsels to your mouth at a cocktail party, but lettuce leaves make a great alternative. Here, ground chicken is flavored with chiles, fresh herbs, and lime for a flavor combination—and serving style—your guests will love.

1½ POUNDS GROUND CHICKEN

2 SHALLOTS, MINCED

2 GARLIC CLOVES, MINCED

1 JALAPEÑO PEPPER, SEEDED AND MINCED

1 TABLESPOON CANOLA OIL

½ CUP CHOPPED FRESH CILANTRO LEAVES

½ CUP CHOPPED FRESH MINT LEAVES

½ CUP CHOPPED FRESH BASIL LEAVES

JUICE OF 1 LIME

1 TABLESPOON FISH SAUCE

1 TEASPOON CHILI PASTE

8 RED LEAF, BOSTON, OR BIBB LETTUCE LEAVES,
    WASHED AND DRIED

1. In a large bowl, stir together the chicken, shallots, garlic, and jalapeño.

2. In a large skillet, heat the oil over medium-high heat and then add the chicken mixture. Cook, stirring and breaking apart the meat with a spatula, until the chicken is cooked through but not browned, 3 or 4 minutes. Remove from the heat.

3. In a medium bowl, stir together the cilantro, mint, basil, lime juice, fish sauce, and chili paste.

continued ▶

4. Add the herb mixture to the chicken mixture and stir to combine well. Transfer to a serving bowl and let cool for several minutes before serving to prevent the lettuce leaves from wilting.

5. Serve the ground meat alongside lettuce leaves, instructing diners to scoop some of the meat into a lettuce leaf, roll it up like a mini burrito, and enjoy.

Spicy Garlic Shrimp

SERVES 8

Simple, spicy, and garlicky, this is a great finger food to serve at a cocktail party or while watching a game. Shrimp is low in calories and full of protein. Garlic and cayenne are said to have veritable superpowers when it comes to keeping you healthy, including lowering your risk of heart disease and cancer.

24 LARGE SHRIMP, PEELED AND DEVEINED, TAILS LEFT ON
4 GARLIC CLOVES, MINCED
½ TEASPOON SALT
⅛ TO ¼ TEASPOON CAYENNE

1. Preheat the broiler.

2. In a shallow baking dish, toss the shrimp with the garlic, salt, and cayenne. Spread the shrimp out in a single layer and broil for 2 to 3 minutes. Turn the shrimp over and broil until they are pink and cooked through, another 2 to 3 minutes.

3. Transfer to a platter and serve immediately with lots of napkins and a bowl for discarding the tails.

Classic Crab Cakes with Red Pepper Aioli

MAKES 8 CAKES

Crab cakes can be a delicious everyday meal or an elegant appetizer for a special occasion. These are quick and easy to make, low in fat and sodium, and full of flavorful herbs and spices and a squeeze of lime.

CRAB CAKES:

½ CUP PANKO BREADCRUMBS

1 LARGE WHOLE EGG PLUS 1 LARGE EGG WHITE, LIGHTLY BEATEN

2 SCALLIONS, THINLY SLICED

2 TABLESPOONS FINELY CHOPPED RED BELL PEPPER

2 TABLESPOONS MINCED FRESH PARSLEY

1 TABLESPOON MAYONNAISE

JUICE OF ½ LIME

1 TEASPOON OLD BAY SEASONING

1 TEASPOON SALT

½ TEASPOON GROUND BLACK PEPPER

9 OUNCES LUMP CRABMEAT

COOKING SPRAY

AIOLI:

¼ CUP PLAIN NONFAT GREEK YOGURT

2 TABLESPOONS MAYONNAISE

¼ CUP ROASTED RED BELL PEPPER (FROM A JAR, PACKED IN WATER), DRAINED, SEEDED, AND MINCED

To make crab cakes:

1. In a large bowl, combine the breadcrumbs, whole egg and egg white, scallions, bell pepper, parsley, mayonnaise, lime juice, Old Bay Seasoning, salt, and black pepper and stir to mix well. With your hands, gently fold in the crabmeat, being careful not to break up the large pieces. Shape into 8 patties and refrigerate for 30 to 60 minutes.

2. Preheat the oven to 400°F and spray a large baking sheet with cooking spray.

3. Arrange the chilled crab cakes on the baking sheet and spray lightly with cooking spray. Bake until golden brown on the bottom, about 10 minutes; then flip the crab cakes over and continue baking until golden brown on the other side, another 10 minutes.

4. While the crab cakes are baking, make the aioli in a small bowl by combining the yogurt, mayonnaise, and roasted red pepper and stirring to combine well.

5. Serve the crab cakes hot, garnished with a dollop of the aioli.

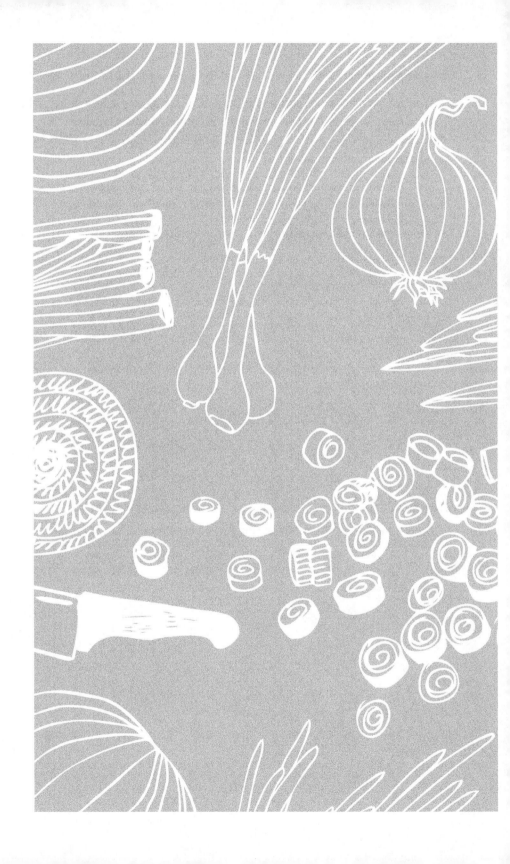

CHAPTER 7

Soups, Salads, and Sandwiches

Roasted Butternut Squash Soup with Apple, Sage, and Gorgonzola

SERVES 4

With its gorgeous orange hue, butternut squash makes a beautiful soup. Roasting it along with the shallots brings out the natural sweetness of both vegetables. A bit of applesauce makes this soup just sweet enough to be a great backdrop for savory sage and salty Gorgonzola cheese.

4 CUPS CUBED BUTTERNUT SQUASH, FRESH OR FROZEN

2 MEDIUM SHALLOTS, DICED

2 TABLESPOONS OLIVE OIL

½ TEASPOON SALT

½ TEASPOON GROUND BLACK PEPPER

4 CUPS CHICKEN BROTH

1 CUP UNSWEETENED APPLESAUCE

3 OUNCES GORGONZOLA, CRUMBLED

1 TABLESPOON MINCED FRESH SAGE

1. Preheat the oven to 400°F.

2. On a large baking sheet, toss together the squash, shallots, olive oil, salt, and pepper. Roast until the squash is very soft and browned in spots, about 45 minutes.

3. Transfer the roasted vegetables to a large stockpot, stir in the broth, and bring to a boil over medium-high heat. Remove the pot from the heat and puree the soup using an immersion blender or in batches using a countertop blender.

4. Stir in the applesauce and reheat the soup over medium heat. Serve the soup hot, garnished with the gorgonzola and sage.

Fennel Soup with Greens

SERVES 6 TO 8

Fennel is a great source of fiber as well as antioxidants and vitamin C. Its slightly exotic flavor makes an alluring base for this quick pureed vegetable soup.

2 TABLESPOONS OLIVE OIL

2 LARGE FENNEL BULBS, TRIMMED AND CHOPPED

2 MEDIUM LEEKS (WHITE AND LIGHT-GREEN PARTS ONLY), CHOPPED

2 SHALLOTS, CHOPPED

1 TABLESPOON CHOPPED FRESH THYME

½ TEASPOON SALT

2 CUPS CHICKEN BROTH

1 CUP WATER

8 OUNCES FRESH SPINACH

¼ TEASPOON GROUND BLACK PEPPER

½ CUP PLAIN LOW-FAT GREEK YOGURT

1 TEASPOON GRATED LEMON ZEST

1 TEASPOON FRESHLY SQUEEZED LEMON JUICE

PINCH OF CAYENNE

1. In a large stockpot, heat the oil over medium heat. Add the fennel, leeks, shallots, thyme, and salt. Cook, covered, until the fennel has softened, about 10 minutes.

2. Add the broth and water, cover again, reduce the heat to low, and simmer for 12 minutes more.

3. Add the spinach and pepper and stir until the spinach is wilted. Remove from the heat, and then puree using an immersion blender or in batches using a countertop blender.

4. In a small bowl, stir together the yogurt, lemon zest, lemon juice, and cayenne.

5. Reheat the soup, if needed, and serve garnished with a dollop of the yogurt mixture.

Smoky Red Lentil Soup

SERVES 4

Red lentils make a beautiful-hued soup. With the addition of tomatoes, paprika, and turmeric, this version is particularly stunning. Quick cooking, full of fiber, and delicious, lentils are an excellent and inexpensive source of vegetarian protein. This spicy soup gets better with time, so make it a day or two ahead if you are able, or make a double batch and eat the leftovers all week.

1 TABLESPOON OLIVE OIL

1 MEDIUM ONION, DICED

2 GARLIC CLOVES, MINCED

2 TEASPOONS GROUND CUMIN

2 TEASPOONS SMOKED PAPRIKA

1 TEASPOONS SWEET PAPRIKA

1 TEASPOON GROUND TURMERIC

1 TEASPOON SALT

¼ TEASPOON GROUND CINNAMON

2 MEDIUM CARROTS, PEELED AND SLICED

7 CUPS VEGETABLE OR CHICKEN BROTH

1½ CUPS DRIED RED LENTILS

1 (14.5-OUNCE) CAN DICED TOMATOES, UNDRAINED

JUICE OF 1 LEMON

LEMON WEDGES

¼ CUP MINCED FRESH PARSLEY

1. In a large stockpot, heat the olive oil over medium-high heat. Add the onion and garlic and sauté, stirring frequently, until the onion is soft, about 5 minutes.

2. Stir in the cumin, smoked paprika, sweet paprika, turmeric, salt, and cinnamon and cook, stirring, for 1 minute.

3. Add the carrots, broth, lentils, and tomatoes along with their juice. Bring to a boil, reduce the heat to medium-low, and simmer, uncovered, until the lentils are soft, 30 to 35 minutes.

4. Just before serving, stir in the lemon juice. Serve hot, garnished with lemon wedges and a generous sprinkling of parsley.

Vegetarian Quinoa Chili

SERVES 6

Nutritionists love quinoa, and for good reason. This great-tasting whole grain is full of protein and fiber and has a low glycemic index. It's a superb low-fat alternative to rice or couscous. Here it's paired with chiles and beans in a flavorful vegetarian chili. Garnish it with grated cheese, sour cream, diced avocados, salsa, minced cilantro, or all of the above.

1 TABLESPOON OLIVE OIL

1 SMALL ONION, CHOPPED

2 GARLIC CLOVES, MINCED

2 CELERY STALKS, DICED

1 LARGE CARROT, PEELED AND DICED

1 BELL PEPPER (ANY COLOR), SEEDED AND DICED

2 JALAPEÑO PEPPERS, SEEDED AND DICED

2 TABLESPOONS CHILI POWDER

1 TABLESPOON GROUND CUMIN

2 (15-OUNCE) CANS PINTO BEANS, RINSED AND DRAINED

1 (28-OUNCE) CAN DICED TOMATOES, DRAINED

1 (15-OUNCE) CAN TOMATO SAUCE

2 CUPS COOKED QUINOA

1. In a large stockpot, heat the olive oil over medium-high heat. Add the onion and garlic and cook, stirring frequently, until the onion is soft, about 5 minutes. Add the celery, carrot, bell pepper, and jalapeños and cook, stirring occasionally, until the vegetables are tender, about 10 minutes. Stir in the chili powder and cumin and cook for 30 seconds more.

2. Add the beans, tomatoes, tomato sauce, and quinoa. Reduce the heat to medium-low, cover, and simmer for 30 minutes. Serve hot.

White Bean and Greens Soup with Sausage

SERVES 6 TO 8

White beans are another excellent source of protein, fiber, and antioxidants. A hefty serving of kale adds even more essential vitamins, minerals, fiber, and anti-oxidants. This hearty soup makes a perfect meal for a cold evening.

2 TABLESPOONS OLIVE OIL

1 MEDIUM ONION, DICED

2 GARLIC CLOVES, MINCED

2 CELERY STALKS, SLICED

2 MEDIUM CARROTS, PEELED AND SLICED

8 OUNCES SPANISH-STYLE CHORIZO OR ANDOUILLE SAUSAGE, DICED

1 BUNCH KALE, CHOPPED

¾ TEASPOON SALT

½ TEASPOON GROUND BLACK PEPPER

4 CUPS CHICKEN BROTH

1 (14.5-OUNCE) CAN DICED TOMATOES, UNDRAINED

1 (15-OUNCE) CAN WHITE BEANS, SUCH AS CANNELLINI OR GREAT
NORTHERN, RINSED AND DRAINED

1. In a large stockpot, heat the oil over medium-high heat. Add the onion and garlic and cook, stirring frequently, until the onion is soft, about 5 minutes.

2. Add the celery, carrots, and sausage and cook, stirring occasionally, for 3 minutes more. Stir in the kale, salt, and pepper.

3. Add the broth, tomatoes along with their juice, and beans and bring to a boil. Reduce the heat to medium-low and simmer, covered, until the vegetables are soft, 15 to 20 minutes. Serve hot.

Beef and Porcini Mushroom Soup

SERVES 6 TO 8

This soup gets better with time. If you can, make it a day ahead so that the flavors can develop overnight. It's meaty and rich, making it a great winter night's meal.

2 TABLESPOONS OLIVE OIL

1½- TO 2-POUND CROSS-CUT MEATY BEEF SHANK BONE

1½ POUNDS BONELESS BEEF CHUCK, CUT INTO ½-INCH CUBES

SALT AND GROUND BLACK PEPPER TO TASTE

2 BAY LEAVES

2 TABLESPOONS CHOPPED FRESH THYME, DIVIDED

2 MEDIUM ONIONS, CHOPPED

4 LARGE CELERY STALKS, DICED

6 CUPS BEEF BROTH

1 (14.5-OUNCE) CAN DICED TOMATOES, UNDRAINED

1 LARGE CARROT, PEELED AND DICED

1 LARGE PARSNIP, PEELED AND DICED

1 OUNCE DRIED PORCINI MUSHROOMS, BROKEN INTO SMALL PIECES

1. In large stockpot, heat the oil over medium-high heat. Add the bone and meat, sprinkle with salt and pepper, and cook, stirring frequently, until the meat is browned on all sides and the juices have mostly evaporated.

2. Add the bay leaves and 1½ tablespoons of the thyme and cook, stirring, for 1 minute. Stir in the onions and celery and cook, stirring, until the vegetables have begun to soften, about 3 minutes. Add the broth, tomatoes along with their juice, carrot, parsnip, and mushrooms. Bring to a boil, and then reduce the heat to medium-low and cook, covered, until the meat is very tender, 1 hour to 1 hour and 15 minutes.

3. Discard the bone and bay leaves. Serve immediately, garnished with the remaining ½ tablespoon thyme, or cover and refrigerate overnight and reheat before serving.

Asparagus and Edamame Salad with Citrus Vinaigrette

SERVES 4

Asparagus heralds the onset of spring and brings with it all sort of healing and protective properties. It's a great source of fiber, antioxidants, vitamins, and the mineral chromium, which enhances insulin's ability to transport glucose to the body's cells. Bright green edamame, too, come loaded with fiber, vitamins, and minerals, as well as a good dose of protein. These two bright-spring-green veggies costar in this lemony salad studded with crunchy, bright-pink radishes and sprinkled with salty Parmesan cheese.

ZEST AND JUICE OF 1 LEMON
1 TABLESPOON WHITE WINE VINEGAR
1 TEASPOON DIJON MUSTARD
1 TEASPOON HONEY
½ TEASPOON SALT
¼ TEASPOON GROUND BLACK PEPPER
3 TABLESPOONS OLIVE OIL
1 POUND ASPARAGUS, WOODY ENDS SNAPPED OFF AND DISCARDED
2 CUPS SHELLED FROZEN EDAMAME, THAWED
½ BUNCH RADISHES (ABOUT 4 OUNCES), HALVED AND THINLY SLICED
6 HANDFULS BABY ARUGULA
¼ CUP (ABOUT 1 OUNCE) GRATED PARMESAN CHEESE

1. To make the dressing, in a small bowl, whisk together the lemon zest and juice, vinegar, mustard, honey, salt, and pepper. Whisk in the olive oil until the dressing is well combined and emulsified. Set aside.

2. Slice the asparagus on the diagonal as thin as possible. In a medium bowl, combine the asparagus, edamame, and radishes. Drizzle about three-quarters of the dressing over them and toss to coat well.

3. In a medium bowl, toss the arugula with the remaining dressing and toss to coat. Arrange the arugula on 4 salad plates, top with the asparagus mixture, and serve immediately, sprinkled with the Parmesan cheese.

Warm Spinach Salad with Thai Peanut Dressing

SERVES 4

In addition to being one of the most versatile greens around, spinach helps protect against cancer as well as inflammatory, cardiovascular, and bone problems. Peanuts are a great source of monounsaturated fats, vitamin E, niacin, folate, and manganese—all known to promote heart health. They also deliver high doses of resveratrol, the antioxidant that gives red wine its heart-healthy reputation.

⅓ CUP ALL-NATURAL, NO-SUGAR-ADDED PEANUT BUTTER

¼ CUP UNSEASONED RICE VINEGAR

3 TABLESPOONS CANOLA OIL

3 TABLESPOONS REDUCED-SODIUM SOY SAUCE

3 TABLESPOONS HONEY

3 GARLIC CLOVES, MINCED

1 TABLESPOON GRATED FRESH GINGER

1 TEASPOON TOASTED SESAME OIL

½ TEASPOON CHILI PASTE OR SRIRACHA SAUCE

½ TEASPOON SALT

COOKING SPRAY

12 CUPS FRESH SPINACH LEAVES

½ CUP LIGHTLY SALTED ROASTED PEANUTS, CHOPPED

1. To make the dressing, in a small bowl, stir together the peanut butter, vinegar, canola oil, soy sauce, honey, garlic, ginger, sesame oil, chili paste or Sriracha sauce, and salt until well combined. Set aside.

2. Heat a large skillet over high heat and spray it with cooking spray. Add the spinach and cook, stirring, just until the spinach begins to wilt. Remove from the heat and immediately transfer to a serving platter.

3. Drizzle the dressing over the spinach, sprinkle with the peanuts, and serve.

Roasted Vegetable Salad with Cumin Vinaigrette

SERVES 4

Roasting vegetables brings out their natural sweetness. This dish is almost like a deconstructed ratatouille. It's delicious, full of an array of healthy veggies, and simple to make. The pumpkin seed garnish provides a nice crunch and may help with insulin regulation.

SALAD:

1 MEDIUM EGGPLANT, PEELED AND DICED

6 TO 8 ROMA TOMATOES, CUT INTO WEDGES

2 MEDIUM CARROTS, PEELED AND CUT INTO SMALL STICKS

1 RED OR YELLOW BELL PEPPER, SEEDED AND SLICED

2 TABLESPOONS OLIVE OIL

1 TEASPOON SALT

½ TEASPOON GROUND BLACK PEPPER

VINAIGRETTE:

2 TABLESPOONS PUMPKIN SEEDS, TOASTED

3 TABLESPOONS RED WINE VINEGAR

1 TEASPOON SWEET PAPRIKA

½ TEASPOON GROUND CUMIN

½ TEASPOON SALT

1 GARLIC CLOVE, MINCED

1 BUNCH FRESH FLAT-LEAF PARSLEY, CHOPPED

6 TABLESPOONS OLIVE OIL

1. Preheat the oven to 400°F.

2. On a large rimmed baking sheet, toss the eggplant, tomatoes, carrots, and bell pepper with the olive oil. Spread the vegetables out in a single layer, sprinkle with the salt and black pepper, and roast until they are tender and beginning to brown, about 40 minutes.

3. To make the dressing, in a small bowl, combine the vinegar, paprika, cumin, salt, garlic, and parsley. Whisk in the olive oil until the dressing is well combined and emulsified.

4. When the vegetables have finished roasting, transfer them to a large bowl. Drizzle the vinaigrette over them and toss to coat well. Cover and refrigerate for at least an hour. Serve cold or at room temperature, garnished with the toasted pumpkin seeds.

Soba Noodle Salad with Shrimp and Ginger

SERVES 4

Soba noodles are made with buckwheat flour, which gives them a distinctive, pleasant flavor and infuses them with much more protein and fiber than noodles made from refined wheat flour.

2 TEASPOONS FINELY GRATED FRESH GINGER, DIVIDED

⅓ CUP MIRIN (RICE WINE), DIVIDED

2 TABLESPOONS FRESHLY SQUEEZED LIME JUICE, DIVIDED

1 TABLESPOON REDUCED-SODIUM SOY SAUCE, DIVIDED

1 POUND SHRIMP, PEELED AND DEVEINED

6 OUNCES DRIED SOBA NOODLES

6 OUNCES SNOW PEAS, TRIMMED

2 TEASPOONS TOASTED SESAME OIL, DIVIDED

2 TABLESPOONS PICKLED GINGER, MINCED

PINCH OF SUGAR

COOKING SPRAY

½ MEDIUM CUCUMBER, PEELED AND DICED

1 BUNCH FRESH CILANTRO, CHOPPED

1. In a large bowl, whisk together the fresh ginger and about half each of the mirin, lime juice, and soy sauce. Add the shrimp and toss to coat. Cover and refrigerate for 20 minutes.

2. While the shrimp is marinating, bring a large pot of water to boil and cook the noodles according to the package directions, adding the snow peas for the last 2 minutes of cooking to blanch them. Drain the noodles and snow peas and transfer them to a large bowl. Drizzle 1 teaspoon of the sesame oil over the noodles and toss to coat.

3. In a small bowl, whisk together the pickled ginger, sugar, and the remaining mirin, lime juice, soy sauce, and sesame oil.

4. Spray a nonstick skillet with cooking spray and heat it over high heat. Add the shrimp and cook, stirring, until they are pink and cooked through, 2 to 3 minutes. Remove from the heat and let cool slightly.

5. Add the cucumber to the noodle mixture and drizzle half of the dressing over the top. Toss to coat well. Divide the noodle mixture among 4 serving bowls and top them with the shrimp and a drizzle of the remaining dressing. Garnish with cilantro and serve.

Steak Salad with Blue Cheese Dressing

SERVES 4

Steak provides a good dose of iron and protein. Flank steak is a lean cut that's perfect for grilling. This quick, easy salad delivers lots of flavor and will satisfy your yearnings for a delicious piece of red meat.

1 (1-POUND) FLANK STEAK, TRIMMED

1 TABLESPOON OLIVE OIL

1 TEASPOON SALT, DIVIDED

½ TEASPOON GROUND BLACK PEPPER

¾ CUP BUTTERMILK

¼ CUP CRUMBLED BLUE CHEESE

½ TEASPOON WORCESTERSHIRE SAUCE

⅛ TEASPOON HOT PEPPER SAUCE

4 SMALL HEADS BIBB LETTUCE, HALVED LENGTHWISE, OR 2 SMALL
    HEADS BOSTON LETTUCE, QUARTERED LENGTHWISE

¼ CUP TOASTED PECAN HALVES, COARSELY CHOPPED

2 TABLESPOONS MINCED FRESH CHIVES

1. Preheat a grill to medium-high heat.

2. Brush the steak on both sides with olive oil, and then sprinkle with ¾ teaspoon of the salt and the black pepper.

3. Grill the steak, turning once, until the desired degree of doneness has been achieved, about 8 minutes per side for medium-rare. Transfer the steak to a cutting board and let rest for 10 minutes.

4. To make the dressing, in a small bowl, stir together the buttermilk, blue cheese, Worcestershire, hot pepper sauce, and remaining ¼ teaspoon salt.

5. When the meat has rested for 10 minutes, cut it across the grain into ¼-inch-thick slices.

6. Divide the lettuce evenly among 4 plates. Arrange the steak decoratively on top of the lettuce. Drizzle the dressing over the top and sprinkle with the pecans. Serve immediately, garnished with chives.

Greek Salad Sandwich

SERVES 4

Nutty, buttery chickpeas are loaded with fiber and protein. Here they serve as a base for a delicious Greek salad that is perfect for stuffing into whole-wheat pitas for a healthy lunch.

1 (15-OUNCE) CAN CHICKPEAS, RINSED AND DRAINED

3 OUNCES FETA CHEESE, CRUMBLED

½ MEDIUM CUCUMBER, PEELED, SEEDED, AND DICED

1 MEDIUM BELL PEPPER (ANY COLOR), SEEDED AND DICED

1 LARGE TOMATO, SEEDED AND DICED

¼ CUP DICED RED ONION

2 TABLESPOONS MINCED FRESH PARSLEY

2 TABLESPOONS FRESHLY SQUEEZED LEMON JUICE

1 TABLESPOON OLIVE OIL

1 TEASPOON DRIED OREGANO

¾ TEASPOON SALT

½ TEASPOON GROUND BLACK PEPPER

4 WHOLE-WHEAT PITA BREADS, WARMED

2 CUPS SHREDDED ROMAINE LETTUCE

1. In a large bowl, gently mash the chickpeas with a fork, until all the beans are slightly crushed. Add the cheese, cucumber, bell pepper, tomato, onion, and parsley and toss to combine. Add the lemon juice, olive oil, oregano, salt, and black pepper and stir to mix.

2. Cut the pita breads in half and stuff the salad mixture into each half. Top each half with a handful of shredded lettuce and serve.

Mediterranean Tuna Salad Sandwiches

SERVES 2

Low-calorie tuna is a great choice when you want a healthy lunch in a hurry. Tuna can be high in mercury, though, so limit yourself to no more than one or two servings a week. This version is full of surprises, including olives, artichoke hearts, and capers.

1 (6-OUNCE) CAN WATER-PACKED TUNA, DRAINED

1 ROMA TOMATO, CHOPPED

4 MARINATED ARTICHOKE HEARTS, DRAINED AND CHOPPED

2 TABLESPOONS MINCED RED ONION

2 TABLESPOONS CHOPPED PITTED KALAMATA OLIVES

1 TABLESPOON MAYONNAISE

1 TEASPOON CAPERS, RINSED AND CHOPPED

1 TEASPOON FRESHLY SQUEEZED LEMON JUICE

½ TEASPOON SALT

¼ TEASPOON GROUND BLACK PEPPER

4 SLICES WHOLE-WHEAT SOURDOUGH BREAD, TOASTED

4 CRISP LETTUCE LEAVES, SUCH AS ROMAINE OR BIBB

1. In a medium bowl, flake the tuna with a fork. Add the tomato, artichoke hearts, onion, olives, mayonnaise, capers, lemon juice, salt, and pepper and mix well with a fork.

2. Divide the tuna mixture between two of the slices of bread, spreading it in an even layer. Top with the lettuce leaves and then the remaining slices of bread. Cut each sandwich in half diagonally and serve.

Chicken Pesto Wraps

SERVES 4

Chicken breast is a great high-protein backdrop for the garlic-and-basil flavors of pesto. Sun-dried tomatoes add an intense dose of umami flavor, while fresh tomatoes keep the whole thing tasting light and fresh.

COOKING SPRAY

2 BONELESS, SKINLESS CHICKEN BREASTS, HALVED CROSSWISE

½ TEASPOON SALT

¼ TEASPOON GROUND BLACK PEPPER

¼ CUP PESTO

4 SUN-DRIED TOMATOES (DRAINED IF PACKED IN OIL), MINCED

4 WHOLE-WHEAT TORTILLAS, WARMED

4 SLICES FRESH MOZZARELLA CHEESE

1 LARGE FRESH TOMATO, CUT INTO THIN WEDGES

4 ROMAINE LETTUCE LEAVES

1. Preheat a nonstick skillet over medium high-heat and spray it with cooking spray. Sprinkle the salt and pepper over the chicken breasts and add the chicken breasts to the pan. Cook until the chicken begins to brown and is cooked through, 4 to 5 minutes per side.

2. Dice the chicken and toss it in a medium bowl with the pesto and sun-dried tomatoes.

3. Divide the chicken mixture evenly among the tortillas, and then top each with a slice of the cheese, a few tomato wedges, and a lettuce leaf. Roll up the wraps, cut in half on the diagonal, and serve.

Ham and Brie Sandwiches with Apple

SERVES 2

Chilling the Brie makes it easier to slice. This is a great lunchbox sandwich because by the time you eat it, the cheese will be a creamy room temperature.

4 SLICES SPROUTED MULTIGRAIN BREAD

2 TABLESPOONS DIJON MUSTARD

6 OUNCES SLICED DELI HAM

3 OUNCES BRIE, CHILLED AND THINLY SLICED

1 GRANNY SMITH OR OTHER TART GREEN APPLE, CORED AND
    THINLY SLICED

1 CUP SALAD GREENS

1. Spread 2 slices of bread with the mustard. Top each with half of the ham, half of the Brie, half of the apple, and half of the salad greens.

2. Place the remaining 2 slices of bread on top of the sandwiches. Slice each sandwich in half diagonally and serve or wrap up and tuck into your lunchbox.

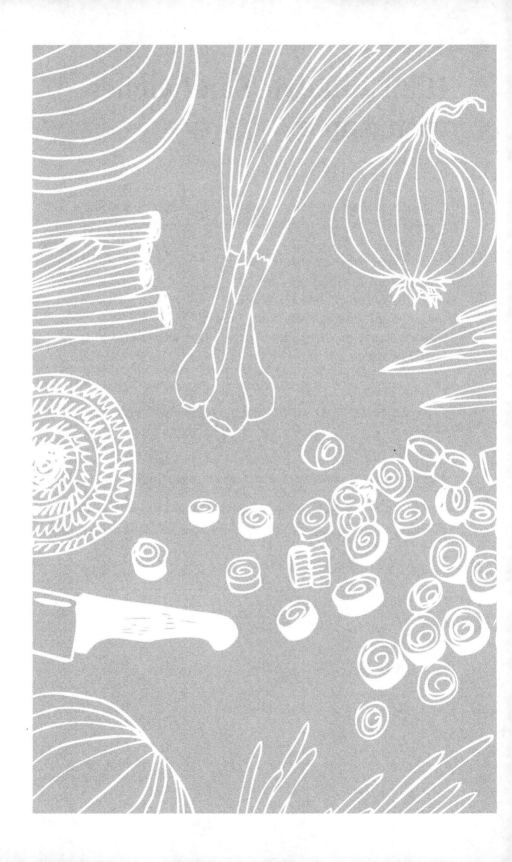

CHAPTER 8

Side Dishes

Maple-Roasted Butternut Squash

SERVES 4

Butternut squash is one of those near-perfect foods; it's beautiful, easy to cook, delicious, and loaded with health-enhancing fiber, minerals, and vitamin A. Sweetened with a touch of maple syrup, this simple side dish makes a great partner for roasted turkey, grilled steak, or white beans stewed with garlic. (Pumpkin is quite similar to butternut squash in flavor and texture, so feel free to substitute it for the squash in this recipe.)

3 CUPS CUBED BUTTERNUT SQUASH, FRESH OR FROZEN

2 TABLESPOONS MAPLE SYRUP

2 TABLESPOONS OLIVE OIL

2 TABLESPOONS CHOPPED FRESH THYME

¾ TEASPOON SALT

½ TEASPOON GROUND BLACK PEPPER

½ TEASPOON GROUND ALLSPICE

1. Preheat the oven to 400°F.

2. On a large rimmed baking sheet, toss the squash with the maple syrup and olive oil. Spread in a single layer and sprinkle with the thyme, salt, pepper, and allspice.

3. Roast until the squash is tender and beginning to brown in places, about 30 minutes. Serve hot.

Quinoa 'n' Cheese

SERVES 4

If you've been missing good old cheesy, starchy mac and cheese, you're in luck. This quinoa-based version has more protein, more fiber, and fewer refined carbs, but it's just as delicious. The added broccoli gives it a bit of green veggie goodness. For an even healthier version, use reduced-fat cheese.

COOKING SPRAY

2 CUPS SMALL BROCCOLI FLORETS

2 LARGE EGGS

1 CUP 1 PERCENT MILK

1½ CUPS GRATED SHARP CHEDDAR CHEESE

2 GARLIC CLOVES, MINCED

1 TEASPOON SALT

6 CUPS COOKED QUINOA

1 CUP WHOLE-WHEAT BREADCRUMBS

1. Preheat the oven to 350°F and spray a 9-by-13-inch baking dish with cooking spray.

2. Bring a medium saucepan of water to a boil and blanch the broccoli until just tender, about 1 minute. Drain in a colander.

3. In a large bowl, whisk the eggs and milk until well combined. Add the cheese, garlic, and salt. Stir in the quinoa and broccoli and mix well. Transfer to the prepared baking dish.

4. Spread the breadcrumbs evenly over the top and bake until bubbling, and lightly browned on top, 30 to 35 minutes. Serve hot.

Smashed Garlicky White Beans with Rosemary

SERVES 6

This creamy bean dish is a welcome substitute for mashed potatoes. It's full of garlicky flavor and offers the same creamy texture as those scrumptious potatoes, but instead of being a pile of fat-laden simple carbs, this version is packed with protein and fiber. Serve it alongside roasted meats or anytime you'd normally offer mashed potatoes.

2 TABLESPOONS OLIVE OIL

2 GARLIC CLOVES, PEELED BUT LEFT WHOLE

2 TEASPOONS MINCED FRESH ROSEMARY

2 (15-OUNCE) CANS CANNELLINI BEANS, RINSED AND DRAINED

¼ CUP CHICKEN OR VEGETABLE BROTH

2 TABLESPOONS GRATED PARMESAN CHEESE

SALT AND GROUND BLACK PEPPER TO TASTE

1. In a large skillet, heat the olive oil over medium-low heat. Add the garlic cloves and rosemary and cook, stirring occasionally, until the garlic softens and begins to brown, 6 to 8 minutes. Mash the garlic with the back of a wooden spoon.

2. Add the beans and cook, stirring occasionally and mashing with the back of a spoon, until thoroughly heated, about 5 minutes. Add the broth while continuing to mash the beans, mixing in the broth. Transfer to a serving bowl; stir in the cheese, salt, and pepper; and serve hot.

Lemony Roasted Brussels Sprouts

SERVES 6

Brussels sprouts can help protect you against cancer and heart disease. Roasting them is an easy way to caramelize their natural sugars and cook out the bitter edge that many people object to. Of course, a hearty dose of garlic and a splash of lemon do wonders as well.

1½ POUNDS BRUSSELS SPROUTS, TRIMMED AND HALVED LENGTHWISE

3 TABLESPOONS OLIVE OIL

4 GARLIC CLOVES, THINLY SLICED

¾ TEASPOON SALT

½ TEASPOON GROUND BLACK PEPPER

ZEST AND JUICE OF 1 LEMON

3 TABLESPOONS GRATED PARMESAN CHEESE (OPTIONAL)

1. Preheat the oven to 400°F.

2. In a large baking dish, toss the Brussels sprouts with the olive oil, garlic, salt, and pepper. Roast, stirring once halfway through, until they are tender inside and browned and beginning to crisp on the outside, 35 to 40 minutes. If they begin to burn on the bottom before they are cooked through, add ¼ cup or so of water to the pan and stir to scrape up any browned bits from the bottom of the pan.

3. Stir in the lemon zest and juice and top with the grated cheese, if using. Serve hot.

Oven-Roasted Root Veggies with Balsamic Vinegar

This easy dish is a million times healthier than french fries (even the oven-baked kind) and at least as many times more delicious. You can add a wider variety of vegetables, or substitute others, like cauliflower, turnips, red onions, Brussels sprouts, or beets.

1 POUND SWEET POTATOES, PEELED AND CUT INTO 1-INCH CHUNKS

1 POUND CARROTS, PEELED AND CUT INTO 1-INCH CHUNKS

1 POUND PARSNIPS, PEELED AND CUT INTO 1-INCH CHUNKS

2 TABLESPOONS OLIVE OIL

2 TABLESPOONS BALSAMIC VINEGAR

1 TEASPOON SALT

½ TEASPOON GROUND BLACK PEPPER

1. Preheat the oven to 400°F.

2. On a large rimmed baking sheet, toss the vegetables with the oil and vinegar. Sprinkle with the salt and pepper. Roast, stirring once halfway through cooking, until the vegetables are tender and beginning to brown, about 40 minutes. Serve hot.

Sautéed Chard with Pine Nuts and Pancetta

This scrumptious dish is an easy way to make sure you're getting your greens. Serve it alongside roasted meat, poultry, or fish. If pancetta isn't available, substitute bacon. You can also use any nut you like, such as almonds or walnuts, in place of the pine nuts.

2 THIN SLICES (1½ OUNCES) PANCETTA, DICED

2 MEDIUM SHALLOTS, THINLY SLICED

1 POUND SWISS CHARD, TOUGH STEMS REMOVED AND LEAVES CHOPPED

¼ CUP WATER

1 TABLESPOON FRESHLY SQUEEZED LEMON JUICE

2 TABLESPOONS PINE NUTS, TOASTED

¼ TEASPOON GROUND BLACK PEPPER

1. Heat a large, heavy skillet over medium-high heat. Add the pancetta and cook, stirring frequently, until it begins to brown, about 5 minutes. Transfer the pancetta to a paper towel–lined plate.

2. Add the shallots to the pan and cook, stirring frequently, until they soften and begin to brown, about 5 minutes. Stir in the chard, water, and lemon juice and continue to cook until the chard is wilted, about 2 more minutes. Cover the pan and continue cooking until the chard is tender.

3. Remove from the heat, add the pine nuts, pepper, and cooked pancetta to the pan, and stir to mix. Serve immediately.

Brown Rice Pilaf with Fresh Herbs

Many people gravitate toward white rice because it's what they're used to, but in a nutrition competition, brown rice will win hands down every time. That's because the refining process that turns brown rice into white involves stripping the rice grain of its outer hull and bran. And the bran is where most of the nutrients—including selenium, manganese, magnesium, iron, and fiber—are found. Try this flavorful pilaf and you may become a brown rice convert for life.

1 TABLESPOON OLIVE OIL

1 SHALLOT, CHOPPED

1 CUP UNCOOKED LONG-GRAIN BROWN RICE

2½ CUPS CHICKEN OR VEGETABLE BROTH

1 GARLIC CLOVE, MINCED

2 SPRIGS FRESH THYME

1 TEASPOON SALT

3 TABLESPOONS CHOPPED FRESH FLAT-LEAF PARSLEY

2 TABLESPOONS MINCED FRESH CHIVES

1. In a 2-quart saucepan, heat the olive oil over medium heat. Add the shallot and cook, stirring, until softened, about 5 minutes. Add the rice and cook, stirring, until the rice is completely coated with oil.

2. Add the broth, garlic, thyme, and salt. Reduce the heat to medium-low, cover, and cook until the rice is tender, about 45 minutes. Remove from the heat and let sit, covered, for 5 minutes or so.

3. Remove and discard the thyme sprigs, stir in the parsley and chives, and serve.

Mediterranean Braised Green Beans

SERVES 4

Green beans are loaded with antioxidants, including vitamin C and beta-carotene, as well as manganese. This braised version is a healthy alternative to the traditional fat-laden green bean casserole that is popular on holiday tables.

1 TABLESPOON OLIVE OIL

2 GARLIC CLOVES, MINCED

1 POUND FRESH GREEN BEANS, TRIMMED

1 (14.5-OUNCE) CAN DICED TOMATOES, UNDRAINED

10 PITTED KALAMATA OLIVES, COARSELY CHOPPED

2 TABLESPOONS CAPERS, DRAINED

½ TEASPOON SALT

½ TEASPOON GROUND BLACK PEPPER

1. In a large skillet, heat the olive oil over medium heat. Add the garlic and cook, stirring, for about 30 seconds. Stir in the green beans and then the tomatoes (along with their juice), olives, capers, salt, and pepper. Bring to a boil; then reduce the heat to low, cover, and simmer until the beans are just tender, about 20 minutes.

2. Remove the lid, raise the heat to medium, and continue cooking until the liquid has mostly evaporated, about 2 minutes more. Serve hot.

Bulgur with Roasted Vegetables and Fresh Herbs

SERVES 4

Bulgur, if you're not familiar with it, is simply a cracked whole grain of wheat and is the basis of Middle Eastern tabbouleh salads. Because it's a whole grain, it is full of fiber and nutrients, making it a great substitute for refined grains like white rice and pasta. This dish is reminiscent of tabbouleh with its lemony dressing and fresh herbs. Roasted vegetables add even more nutrients and fiber.

1 CUP DRIED BULGUR

¾ TEASPOON SALT, DIVIDED

1 CUP BOILING WATER

2 MEDIUM ZUCCHINI, DICED

2 SWEET ONIONS SUCH AS VIDALIA, DICED

2 CUPS DICED MUSHROOMS

2 CUPS CHERRY TOMATOES, HALVED

3 TABLESPOONS OLIVE OIL, DIVIDED

½ TEASPOON GROUND BLACK PEPPER

3 TABLESPOONS FRESHLY SQUEEZED LEMON JUICE

½ CUP CHOPPED FRESH PARSLEY

½ CUP CHOPPED FRESH MINT

¼ CUP WALNUTS, CHOPPED AND TOASTED

1. Preheat the oven to 375°F.

2. In a large heat-proof bowl, combine the bulgur and ½ teaspoon of the salt. Pour the boiling water over the bulgur, stir, cover tightly, and let sit until the bulgur is tender, about 30 minutes.

3. Meanwhile, toss the zucchini, onions, mushrooms, and tomatoes on a large, rimmed baking sheet with 1 tablespoon of the olive oil. Season with the remaining ¼ teaspoon of salt and the pepper. Spread the vegetables out in a single layer and roast until the vegetables are tender, 25 to 30 minutes.

4. Add the remaining 2 tablespoons olive oil to the bulgur, along with the lemon juice, parsley, and mint. Stir to mix well. Add the roasted vegetables, stir, and serve garnished with the walnuts.

Whole-Wheat Pasta with White Beans

SERVES 4

Using whole-wheat pasta in place of white pasta gives this dish a big boost of fiber and nutrition. And pairing the pasta with beans gives it plenty of protein and even more fiber. Serve this dish alongside roast chicken or as a meal in itself with a crisp green salad.

2 TABLESPOONS OLIVE OIL

1 SMALL ONION, FINELY DICED

1 MEDIUM CARROT, PEELED AND FINELY DICED

1 CELERY STALK, FINELY DICED

2 GARLIC CLOVES, MINCED

2 TABLESPOONS MINCED FRESH PARSLEY

1 TEASPOON SALT

⅛ TEASPOON CRUSHED RED PEPPER FLAKES

2 TABLESPOONS TOMATO PASTE

1½ CUPS WATER, DIVIDED

1 (15-OUNCE) CAN WHITE BEANS, SUCH AS CANNELLINI OR GREAT
  NORTHERN, RINSED AND DRAINED

8 OUNCES DRIED WHOLE-WHEAT PENNE

¼ CUP GRATED PARMESAN CHEESE

1½ TEASPOONS MINCED FRESH ROSEMARY

1. Bring a large pot of water to boil for the pasta.

2. Meanwhile, in a large saucepan, heat 2 tablespoons of the oil over medium heat. Add the onion, carrot, celery, garlic, parsley, salt, and red pepper flakes and cook, stirring occasionally, until the vegetables begin to brown, about 10 minutes. Stir in the tomato paste and continue cooking for another minute, and then add ½ cup of the water and stir to scrape up any browned bits from the bottom of the pan. Reduce the heat to low and simmer until the liquid has mostly evaporated, 6 to 8 minutes. Stir in the beans and the remaining 1 cup water and continue to simmer for 15 minutes more.

3. While the vegetables are cooking, cook the pasta al dente according to the package directions. Drain the pasta, reserving about a cup of the cooking water.

4. Scoop a cup of the bean and vegetable mixture into a food processor and process until smooth. Stir the puree back into the pot with the beans. Add the cooked pasta and a bit of the cooking water and cook, stirring, until the sauce and pasta are well mixed, about 2 minutes. If desired, add more cooking water to thin the sauce. Serve garnished with the Parmesan cheese and rosemary.

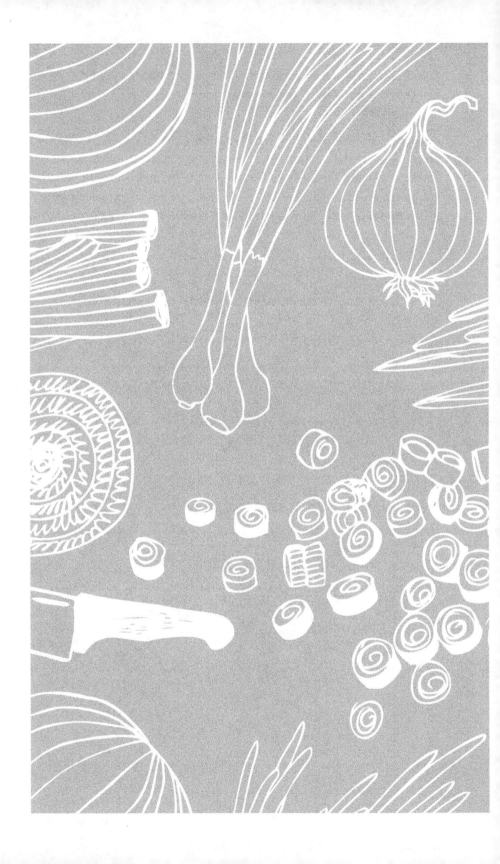

CHAPTER 9

Main Dishes

Summer Vegetable Gratin

This light vegetarian entrée highlights the best of summer produce—ripe, red tomatoes, bright yellow squash, earthy red onions, and fresh herbs—all held together with a light but flavorful cheese sauce.

COOKING SPRAY

5 TEASPOONS OLIVE OIL, DIVIDED

2 MEDIUM RED ONIONS, CHOPPED

1 LARGE RED BELL PEPPER, SEEDED AND CHOPPED

1 POUND YELLOW SQUASH, CUT INTO ¼-INCH-THICK SLICES

2 GARLIC CLOVES, MINCED

1 CUP COOKED QUINOA

½ CUP THINLY SLICED FRESH BASIL, DIVIDED

1½ TEASPOONS CHOPPED FRESH THYME

¾ TEASPOON SALT, DIVIDED

½ TEASPOON GROUND BLACK PEPPER

½ CUP 2 PERCENT MILK

3 OUNCES GRUYÈRE CHEESE, SHREDDED (ABOUT   CUP)

3 LARGE EGGS, LIGHTLY BEATEN

1 LARGE TOMATO, CUT INTO 8 SLICES

1 CUP WHOLE-WHEAT BREADCRUMBS

1. Preheat the oven to 375°F and spray an 11-by-7-inch baking dish with cooking spray.

2. In a large skillet, heat the oil over medium-high heat. Add the onions and cook, stirring, until they begin to soften, about 3 minutes. Add the bell pepper and cook for 2 minutes more. Stir in the squash and garlic and continue to cook, stirring occasionally, for 5 minutes more. Transfer the vegetable mixture to a large bowl and add the quinoa, ¼ cup of the basil, the thyme, ½ teaspoon of the salt, and the black pepper.

3. In a medium bowl, whisk together the milk, cheese, eggs, and remaining ¼ teaspoon salt. Transfer the mixture to the prepared baking dish and lay the tomato slices on top in a single layer. Cover with the breadcrumbs, spritz with a little cooking spray, and bake until the topping is nicely browned, about 40 minutes.

4. Serve hot, garnished with the remaining ¼ cup basil.

Spinach, Chickpea, and Sweet Potato Stew with Coconut Milk

SERVES 4

This quick and hearty stew is comfort food at its best. It's delicious, creamy, and satisfying, and it's also super healthy. This stew has vitamins, minerals, antioxidants, healthy fats, and plenty of fiber to give you sustenance for days.

2 TABLESPOON COCONUT OR CANOLA OIL

1 MEDIUM ONION, CHOPPED

4 GARLIC CLOVES, MINCED

1 TABLESPOON GRATED FRESH GINGER

ZEST OF 1 LEMON

¼ TEASPOON CRUSHED RED PEPPER FLAKES

2 TABLESPOONS TOMATO PASTE

1 (15-OUNCE) CAN CHICKPEAS, RINSED AND DRAINED

2 MEDIUM SWEET POTATOES, PEELED AND DICED

1 (14-OUNCE) CAN UNSWEETENED COCONUT MILK

1 TEASPOON SALT

1 TEASPOON GROUND GINGER

1 POUND BABY SPINACH

¼ CUP CHOPPED FRESH CILANTRO

¼ CUP UNSWEETENED COCONUT FLAKES, TOASTED

1. In a large stockpot, heat the oil over medium-high heat. Add the onion and cook, stirring occasionally, until the onion is softened and beginning to brown, about 5 minutes. Stir in the garlic, fresh ginger, lemon zest, and red pepper flakes and continue to cook, stirring frequently, for 3 minutes more. Stir in the tomato paste and cook for another minute, and then add the chickpeas and sweet potatoes.

2. Raise the heat to high and cook for 3 minutes. Stir in the coconut milk, salt, and ground ginger and heat until simmering. Reduce the heat to low and cook until the sweet potatoes are tender, about 15 minutes. Add the spinach one handful at a time, cooking after each handful until the spinach is wilted before adding another handful, and then cook for a few minutes to ensure that the spinach is cooked and warmed through.

3. Garnish with cilantro and coconut flakes and serve hot.

Veggie Pot Pie

SERVES 8

Pot pie is a true comfort food classic, the kind of dish that fond childhood memories are made of. This version is meat-free and loaded with healthy veggies. The crust is even healthier than the standard type since it's made with whole-wheat pastry flour.

CRUST:

1¼ CUPS WHOLE-WHEAT PASTRY FLOUR

⅛ TEASPOON SALT

7 TABLESPOONS UNSALTED BUTTER, VERY COLD AND CUT INTO PIECES

2 TO 3 TABLESPOONS ICE WATER

FILLING:

1 TABLESPOON UNSALTED BUTTER

2 SMALL FENNEL BULBS, TRIMMED AND DICED

1 SMALL ONION, DICED

2 MEDIUM CARROTS, PEELED AND DICED

12 OUNCES CREMINI OR BUTTON MUSHROOMS, SLICED

1 SMALL SWEET POTATO, PEELED AND DICED

1 TEASPOON SALT

1 TEASPOON GROUND BLACK PEPPER

¼ CUP WHOLE-WHEAT FLOUR

1 CUP MUSHROOM BROTH

1 CUP WHOLE MILK

1 CUP FROZEN BABY GREEN PEAS

2 TEASPOONS MINCED FRESH THYME

1 TABLESPOON WHITE VINEGAR

1 LARGE EGG YOLK WHISKED WITH 2 TEASPOONS WATER
AND A PINCH OF SALT

1. Place the flour and salt in a food processor. Add the butter and pulse until the mixture resembles coarse meal. Add the ice water ½ tablespoon at a time, pulsing between each addition, until the dough just comes together in a ball.

2. Remove the ball of dough from the food processor and pat it into a flat disk. Wrap in plastic wrap and refrigerate for 30 minutes.

3. Preheat the oven to 400°F.

4. In a large stockpot or saucepan, melt the butter over medium heat. Add the fennel, onion, and carrots and cook until the onions begin to soften, about 2 minutes. Add the mushrooms, sweet potato, salt, and pepper and stir to mix. Cook, stirring occasionally, until the mushrooms are soft and most of the liquid has evaporated, 5 to 7 minutes.

5. Sprinkle the flour over the vegetables and stir to mix. Continue to cook, stirring, for 2 more minutes. Stir in the broth and milk and cook, stirring constantly, until the mixture is smooth. Bring to a simmer, reduce the heat to low, and simmer until the sauce begins to thicken, 6 to 8 minutes.

6. Stir in the peas, thyme, and vinegar and remove from the heat. Transfer the mixture to an 8-inch square baking dish or 2-quart casserole dish.

7. Roll out the chilled dough on a lightly floured surface into a 10-inch circle, about ⅛ inch thick.

8. Place the dough over the filling and trim the edges to just about 1 inch wider than the baking dish. Tuck the edges inside the dish and crimp them decoratively. Brush the dough with the egg yolk mixture and cut a few slits in the crust to let steam escape during cooking.

9. Place the baking dish on a baking sheet and bake until the filling is bubbling and the crust is golden brown, 25 to 30 minutes. Let cool for at least 5 minutes before serving. Serve hot.

Seared Trout with Cherry Tomatoes and Bacon

SERVES 4

Here you get all the protein and heart-healthy benefits of trout paired with the smoky flavor of bacon. Serve this dish with quinoa and Lemony Roasted Brussels Sprouts (see page 103).

2 SLICES BACON

1 PINT CHERRY TOMATOES, HALVED

1 GARLIC CLOVE, MINCED

1 TEASPOON GROUND BLACK PEPPER

1 TABLESPOON MINCED FRESH THYME

COOKING SPRAY

1 TEASPOON SALT

4 (6-OUNCE) TROUT FILLETS

4 LEMON WEDGES

1. Heat a medium skillet over medium-high heat. Add the bacon and cook, turning once, until crisp, 5 to 7 minutes. Transfer the bacon strips to a paper towel–lined plate to drain, and then crumble them. Drain off all but about 1 tablespoon of the bacon fat from the pan.

2. Add the cherry tomatoes, garlic, and pepper to the bacon fat in the pan and cook, stirring, until the tomatoes just begin to break down, about 3 minutes. Remove from the heat, and stir in the crumbled bacon and thyme.

3. Spray a large nonstick skillet with cooking spray and heat it over medium-high heat. Sprinkle the salt over the fish fillets and then add them to the pan (you may need to cook the fish in two batches to avoid overcrowding). Cook the fish, turning once, until it is cooked through and flakes easily with a fork, 2 to 3 minutes per side.

4. Transfer the fish fillets to serving plates and serve topped with the tomato mixture and lemon wedges on the side.

Tomato Sauce–Baked Cod with Olives

SERVES 4

Cod is a great low-fat source of protein and delivers heart-healthy omega-3 fatty acids along with other essential vitamins and minerals. Here a rich tomato sauce, loaded with the powerful antioxidant lycopene, bathes the fish in tanginess. Fresh basil, olives, and capers add their intense flavors to the mix.

2 TABLESPOONS OLIVE OIL

3 GARLIC CLOVES, MINCED

1 SMALL BUNCH FRESH BASIL, LEAVES CHOPPED AND STEMS MINCED

1 RED JALAPEÑO PEPPER, HALVED AND SEEDED

1 (28-OUNCE) CAN DICED TOMATOES, UNDRAINED

1 TEASPOON SALT, PLUS MORE FOR THE COD

½ TEASPOON GROUND BLACK PEPPER, PLUS MORE FOR THE COD

1 TEASPOON RED WINE VINEGAR

4 (6-OUNCE) COD FILLETS

1 HANDFUL BLACK OLIVES, PITTED

1 TABLESPOON CAPERS, DRAINED

1. In a large skillet, heat the olive oil over medium heat. Add the garlic, minced basil stems, and jalapeño to the pan and cook, stirring frequently, until the garlic is softened, about 3 minutes.

2. Add the tomatoes along with their juice, salt, and pepper. Bring to a boil, and then reduce the heat to low and simmer for 30 minutes. Remove from the heat and discard the two jalapeño halves. Stir in the vinegar.

3. Preheat the oven to 425°F.

4. Transfer the tomato sauce to a 9-by-13-inch baking dish. Sprinkle the fish fillets with salt and pepper to taste, and then place them on top of the sauce. Scatter the olives, capers, and basil leaves over the top.

5. Bake until the fish is cooked through and flakes easily with a fork, about 15 minutes. Serve immediately.

Spicy Grilled Shrimp Skewers with Cucumber-Cashew Salad

SERVES 4

Healthy, low-calorie, high-protein, quick-cooking shrimp are perfect for grilling. Here they get a spicy rub and are served atop a refreshing cucumber salad to cool the fire. This is an excellent meal for grilling and enjoying outside on a warm summer evening.

CUCUMBER SALAD:

2 MEDIUM CUCUMBERS, PEELED, SEEDED, AND DICED

½ CUP UNSALTED ROASTED CASHEWS, COARSELY CHOPPED

¼ CUP FRESH FLAT-LEAF PARSLEY, CHOPPED

2 SCALLIONS, THINLY SLICED

2 TABLESPOONS OLIVE OIL

1 TABLESPOON FRESHLY SQUEEZED LEMON JUICE

1 TEASPOON SALT

GRILLED SHRIMP SKEWERS:

1 LARGE SERRANO PEPPER, SEEDED AND FINELY MINCED

1 TABLESPOON OLIVE OIL

1 TEASPOON GROUND CUMIN

1 TEASPOON GROUND CHILI POWDER

1 TEASPOON SALT

1 TO 1½ POUNDS PEELED AND DEVEINED SHRIMP

1. Preheat the grill to medium-high and soak 4 wooden skewers in water.

2. To make the salad, in a large bowl, toss together the cucumbers, cashews, parsley, scallions, olive oil, lemon juice, and salt.

3. To make the shrimp, in a large bowl, combine the pepper, olive oil, cumin, chili powder, and salt. Add the shrimp to the bowl and toss to coat with the spice mixture. Thread the shrimp onto the skewers.

4. Grill the shrimp until they are pink and cooked through, about 3 minutes per side.

5. To serve, divide the cucumber salad among 4 serving plates. Top each one with a skewer and serve immediately.

Artichoke-Stuffed Chicken Breasts with Goat Cheese

SERVES 4

Despite their prickly façade, artichokes are full of good-for-you nutrients like fiber, folate, and vitamins C and K. Plus they're one of the most antioxidant-rich foods around. Tangy goat cheese and lemon are perfect flavor partners, and together they turn plain chicken breast into a feast.

1 (6-OUNCE) JAR MARINATED ARTICHOKE HEARTS,
    DRAINED AND CHOPPED
1 (3-OUNCE) PACKAGE HERBED GOAT CHEESE, SOFTENED
2½ TABLESPOONS WHOLE-WHEAT BREADCRUMBS
2 TEASPOONS ITALIAN SEASONING
2 TEASPOONS GRATED LEMON ZEST
½ TEASPOON SALT
¼ TEASPOON GROUND BLACK PEPPER
4 (6-OUNCE) BONELESS, SKINLESS CHICKEN BREAST HALVES
COOKING SPRAY

1. Preheat the oven to 375°F.

2. In a medium bowl, stir together the artichoke hearts, goat cheese, breadcrumbs, Italian seasoning, lemon zest, salt, and pepper.

3. On a sturdy work surface, place one chicken breast on a piece of plastic wrap and cover it with another piece of plastic wrap. Then, using a meat tenderizing mallet or a rolling pin, pound it to an even thickness of about ¼ inch. Repeat with the remaining chicken breasts.

4. Place about 2 tablespoons of the cheese mixture on one end of each of the chicken pieces and roll the chicken up around it. Secure with toothpicks.

5. Coat a large, oven-safe skillet with cooking spray and heat it over medium-high heat. Brown the chicken, about 3 minutes per side. Transfer the skillet to the oven and bake until the chicken is cooked through, about 15 minutes.

Oven-Baked Chicken Legs with Leeks and Onions

SERVES 4

A chicken dish that's easy to toss together in a baking dish and pop in the oven is perfect for busy weeknights and ideal for entertaining. In this mustard-glazed version, whole chicken legs absorb rich flavor from a bed of onions and leeks, and the onions and leeks cook to caramelized deliciousness, incorporating the flavorful juices from the chicken. Serve with a side of sautéed green beans and a scoop of quinoa for a healthy and satisfying meal.

2 MEDIUM ONIONS, THINLY SLICED

2 MEDIUM LEEKS (WHITE AND LIGHT-GREEN PARTS ONLY), THINLY SLICED

4 GARLIC CLOVES, THINLY SLICED

3 TABLESPOONS OLIVE OIL, DIVIDED

2 TEASPOONS FRESH THYME LEAVES

1 TEASPOON SALT

2½ POUNDS BONE-IN, SKINLESS CHICKEN LEG QUARTERS (DRUMSTICKS AND THIGHS)

¼ CUP DIJON MUSTARD

1 SMALL SHALLOT, MINCED

1½ TEASPOONS CHOPPED FRESH ROSEMARY

1 TEASPOON REDUCED-SODIUM SOY SAUCE

¾ TEASPOON GROUND BLACK PEPPER

1. Preheat the oven to 400°F.

2. In a 9-by-13-inch baking dish, combine the onions, leeks, garlic, 2 tablespoons of the olive oil, thyme, and salt and toss to coat the vegetables well. Spread in an even layer. Place the chicken legs on top of the vegetables and bake for 10 minutes.

continued ▶

3. Meanwhile, in a small bowl, whisk together the mustard, shallot, rosemary, soy sauce, and pepper. Add the remaining 1 tablespoon oil and whisk until the mixture is well combined and emulsified.

4. Remove the chicken from the oven and brush the chicken pieces all over with the mustard mixture. Return the pan to the oven and bake until the chicken is cooked through, about 40 minutes more. Serve the chicken legs hot with the onion and leek mixture spooned over the top.

Chicken Curry

Yogurt in the marinade for this spicy curry serves to both flavor and tenderize the meat. In the sauce, the yogurt adds creaminess but not much fat. Serve this dish over steamed brown rice or quinoa, with a side of roasted broccoli or cauliflower or sautéed green beans to round out the meal.

CHICKEN:

1 CUP PLAIN LOW-FAT GREEK YOGURT

1 TABLESPOON MINCED FRESH GINGER

2 TEASPOONS GROUND CUMIN

2 TEASPOONS CHILI POWDER

1 TEASPOON GROUND CINNAMON

1 TEASPOON SALT

½ TEASPOON GROUND BLACK PEPPER

1½ POUNDS BONELESS, SKINLESS CHICKEN BREASTS, CUT INTO
    BITE-SIZED PIECES

SAUCE:

1 TABLESPOON BUTTER

2 GARLIC CLOVES, MINCED

2 RED CHILES, SEEDED AND MINCED

2 TEASPOONS GROUND CUMIN

2 TEASPOONS SWEET PAPRIKA

1 (14.5-OUNCE) CAN DICED TOMATOES, UNDRAINED

1 TEASPOON SALT

½ TEASPOON GROUND BLACK PEPPER

1 CUP PLAIN LOW-FAT GREEK YOGURT

¼ CUP CHOPPED FRESH CILANTRO

continued ▶

To prepare the chicken:

1. In a large bowl, combine the yogurt, ginger, cumin, chili powder, cinnamon, salt, and pepper and stir to mix. Add the chicken and toss to coat well. Cover and let marinate in the refrigerator overnight.

2. Preheat the grill to medium-high heat and soak 4 wooden skewers in water. Remove the chicken pieces from the marinade and thread them onto skewers.

To make the sauce:

1. In a large skillet, melt the butter over medium heat. Add the garlic and chiles and cook, stirring, until they begin to soften and become fragrant, about 2 minutes. Add the cumin and paprika and cook, stirring, for 1 minute. Add the tomatoes along with their juice, salt, and pepper. Continue to cook, stirring and scraping up any browned bits from the bottom of the pan, until the liquid comes to a boil, about 3 minutes. Reduce the heat to low and simmer, uncovered, until the sauce thickens, about 15 minutes.

2. While the sauce is simmering, grill the chicken skewers, turning to cook the pieces evenly, until cooked through, 6 to 8 minutes.

3. Add the grilled chicken and the yogurt to the sauce and simmer, uncovered, for another 10 minutes or so, until the sauce is thick and the chicken is heated through. Serve immediately, garnished with cilantro.

White Chicken Chili

SERVES 4

If you crave the hearty flavor of chili but are intent on keeping excess fat and calories out of your diet, white chicken chili is the dish for you. Garnish this spicy version with diced avocado, fresh salsa, sour cream, shredded cheese, or tortilla chips as desired. Chili is one of those dishes that gets better with time, so consider making a double batch; you can store the extra in a sealed container in the refrigerator for up to 3 days or in the freezer for up to 3 months.

1 TABLESPOON CANOLA OIL

1 ONION, CHOPPED

3 GARLIC CLOVES, MINCED

1 TO 3 JALAPEÑO PEPPERS, SEEDED AND DICED

2 (4-OUNCE) CANS DICED MILD GREEN CHILES, DRAINED

2 TEASPOONS GROUND CUMIN

1½ TEASPOONS GROUND CORIANDER

1 TEASPOON CHILI POWDER

1 TEASPOON DRIED OREGANO

1 TEASPOON SALT

¼ TO ½ TEASPOON GROUND CAYENNE PEPPER

3½ CUPS CHICKEN BROTH

3 CUPS CHOPPED COOKED CHICKEN BREAST

3 (15-OUNCE) CANS WHITE BEANS, SUCH AS CANNELLINI OR GREAT
     NORTHERN, RINSED AND DRAINED

¼ CUP CHOPPED FRESH CILANTRO

1. In a large stockpot, heat the oil over medium heat. Add the onion and garlic and cook, stirring frequently, until the onion is soft, about 5 minutes. Add the jalapeño, green chiles, cumin, coriander, chili powder, oregano, salt, and cayenne. Cook, stirring frequently, until the jalapeño begins to soften, 2 to 3 minutes.

2. Add the broth, chicken, and beans and bring to a boil over medium-high heat. Reduce the heat to medium-low and simmer, uncovered, stirring occasionally, for 15 minutes. Serve hot, garnished with cilantro.

Hoisin Pork and Veggie Stir-Fry

SERVES 4

This classic savory-sweet sauce flavors lean pork tenderloin and veggies for a one-pot meal that's sure to become a favorite. Serve over steamed brown rice for a complete meal.

¼ CUP HOISIN SAUCE

1 TABLESPOON MIRIN (RICE WINE), DRY SHERRY, OR DRY WHITE WINE

5 TEASPOONS TOASTED SESAME OIL, DIVIDED

1 TABLESPOON GRATED FRESH GINGER

2 GARLIC CLOVES, MINCED

1½ POUNDS PORK TENDERLOIN, THINLY SLICED

2 TABLESPOONS SESAME SEEDS

1 MEDIUM SHALLOT, THINLY SLICED

1 CUP SNOW PEAS, THINLY SLICED LENGTHWISE

2 CUPS SHREDDED CHINESE CABBAGE

1 SMALL RED BELL PEPPER, SEEDED AND SLICED INTO MATCHSTICKS

1 TABLESPOON CORNSTARCH MIXED WITH 1 TABLESPOON WATER

4 SCALLIONS, TRIMMED AND THINLY SLICED ON THE DIAGONAL

1. In a large bowl, stir together the hoisin sauce, mirin, 1 tablespoon of the sesame oil, the ginger, and the garlic. Add the pork and toss to coat well. Marinate, covered, in the refrigerator for at least 1 hour or overnight.

2. In a large skillet, toast the sesame seeds over medium heat until they become fragrant, 2 to 3 minutes. Transfer to a bowl and set aside.

3. Remove the pork from the marinade, reserving the marinade.

4. Add the remaining 2 teaspoons sesame oil to the skillet and heat over medium-high heat. Add the shallot and cook, stirring, until it begins to soften,

about 3 minutes. Add the pork, snow peas, cabbage, and bell pepper and cook, stirring, until the vegetables begin to soften, about 3 minutes. Stir in the reserved marinade and bring to a boil. Cook, stirring, until the sauce begins to thicken, about 3 minutes. Add the cornstarch mixture and cook, stirring, until the sauce has thickened, about 2 minutes more. Serve garnished with the scallions and toasted sesame seeds.

Grilled Steak Tacos

SERVES 4

When you hear the words taco *and* steak, *healthy and low-fat are probably not the first things that come to mind. But these grilled steak tacos are both low in fat and good for you. You get lots of iron and protein from the steak, and the salsa, cabbage, and radishes pack in the veggies. You can substitute boneless, skinless chicken breast for the steak for an even lower-fat meal.*

1 TABLESPOON CHILI POWDER

1½ TEASPOONS SALT, DIVIDED

1 TEASPOON BROWN SUGAR

1 TEASPOON GROUND CUMIN

1 TEASPOON DRIED OREGANO

½ TEASPOON GROUND BLACK PEPPER

⅛ TEASPOON GROUND CINNAMON

1 (1-POUND) FLANK STEAK, TRIMMED

2 LARGE TOMATOES, DICED

1 SMALL RED ONION, FINELY DICED

¼ CUP CHOPPED FRESH CILANTRO

1 JALAPEÑO OR SERRANO PEPPER, SEEDED AND FINELY DICED

2 TABLESPOONS FRESHLY SQUEEZED LIME JUICE

1 TEASPOON GRATED LIME ZEST

8 (6-INCH) CORN TORTILLAS

2 CUPS SHREDDED GREEN CABBAGE

4 RADISHES, THINLY SLICED

LIME WEDGES

1. Preheat the grill to medium-high heat and the oven to 350°F.

2. In a small bowl, combine the chili powder, 1 teaspoon of the salt, the brown sugar, cumin, oregano, black pepper, and cinnamon. Rub the spice mixture all over the steak.

3. Grill the steak, turning once, until the desired degree of doneness has been achieved, about 7 minutes per side for medium-rare. Transfer the steak to a cutting board, tent loosely with foil, and let rest for 10 minutes.

4. While the steak is cooking, in a medium bowl, combine the tomatoes, onion, cilantro, jalapeño pepper, lime juice, lime zest, and remaining 1/2 teaspoon salt. Mix well and let stand for 15 minutes or so before serving.

5. Meanwhile, wrap the tortillas in aluminum foil. Heat the tortillas in the oven for about 15 minutes.

6. When the steak has rested, cut it across the grain into 1/4-inch-thick slices.

7. Serve the steak with the warm tortillas, salsa, shredded cabbage, radishes, and lime wedges.

Beef and Broccoli with Soba Noodles

SERVES 4

Soba noodles are made from buckwheat flour, a whole-grain flour that is high in fiber and other nutrients. They have a strong, nutty flavor that stands up well to the hearty flavor of beef.

6 OUNCES DRY SOBA NOODLES

4 CUPS BROCCOLI FLORETS

½ CUP REDUCED-SODIUM SOY SAUCE

⅓ CUP RICE VINEGAR

2 TABLESPOONS FRESHLY GRATED GINGER

1 TABLESPOON TOASTED SESAME OIL

1 TEASPOON SUGAR

½ TEASPOON GROUND BLACK PEPPER

COOKING SPRAY

1 POUND LOIN STEAK, CUT INTO ½-INCH STRIPS

1. Cook the soba noodles according to the package directions.

2. Meanwhile, fill a large pot with a steamer basket with 1 inch of water and bring to a boil. Place the broccoli in the steamer basket, cover, and steam until the broccoli is tender but still bright green, 8 to 10 minutes.

3. In a large bowl, combine the cooked noodles and broccoli.

4. In a small bowl, stir together the soy sauce, rice vinegar, ginger, sesame oil, sugar, and pepper.

5. Spray a large, nonstick skillet with cooking spray and heat it over high heat. Add the beef and cook, stirring frequently, until just cooked through, about 5 minutes. Remove the beef from the pan and keep it warm.

6. Add the sauce mixture to the pan and bring to a boil over high heat. Reduce the heat to low and simmer for 3 or 4 minutes.

7. Divide the broccoli-noodle mixture among 4 serving plates and top each with one-fourth of the meat. Drizzle the sauce over the top and serve immediately.

Spicy Lettuce-Wrapped Beef

SERVES 4

Lean flank steak satisfies that red-meat craving and provides a good dose of iron. This is a fun, do-it-yourself dish for a family dinner or casual dinner party. If you like, serve bowls of additional condiments like chopped fresh herbs, sliced chiles, chili paste, Asian-style pickles, or kimchi.

½ TEASPOON SALT

¼ TEASPOON GROUND BLACK PEPPER

1 POUND FLANK STEAK

½ MEDIUM CUCUMBER, PEELED AND DICED

6 CHERRY TOMATOES, HALVED

1 SMALL SHALLOT, THINLY SLICED

1 TABLESPOON FINELY CHOPPED FRESH MINT

1 TABLESPOON FINELY CHOPPED FRESH BASIL

1 TABLESPOON FINELY CHOPPED FRESH CILANTRO

2 TABLESPOONS REDUCED-SODIUM SOY SAUCE

2 TABLESPOONS FRESHLY SQUEEZED LIME JUICE

1 TABLESPOON BROWN SUGAR

½ TEASPOON CRUSHED RED PEPPER FLAKES

1 HEAD BIBB LETTUCE, LEAVES SEPARATED AND RINSED

1. Preheat the grill to medium-high heat

2. Sprinkle the salt and black pepper over both sides of the steak.

3. Grill the steak until the desired degree of doneness has been achieved, about 7 minutes per side for medium-rare. Transfer the steak to a cutting board, tent loosely with foil, and let rest for 5 to 10 minutes. Then cut the steak across the grain into ¼-inch-thick slices.

4. In a large bowl, combine the sliced steak, cucumber, tomatoes, shallot, mint, basil, and cilantro. In a small bowl, whisk together the soy sauce, lime

juice, brown sugar, and crushed red pepper. Pour this mixture over the steak mixture and toss to coat.

5. To serve, instruct diners to scoop some of the meat into a lettuce leaf, wrap it up like a burrito, and enjoy.

Lamb Chops with Minted Pea Puree

SERVES 4

Both peas and lamb symbolize the arrival of spring, making them a perfect match. Lamb is loaded with iron and zinc, while peas contain both omega-3 and omega-6 fatty acids, which help your body absorb important nutrients.

4 TEASPOONS OLIVE OIL, DIVIDED

3 GARLIC CLOVES, MINCED

2 CUPS FROZEN PEAS, THAWED

¾ CUP WATER, PLUS MORE AS NEEDED

¾ TEASPOON SALT, DIVIDED

½ TEASPOON GROUND BLACK PEPPER

8 LAMB LOIN CHOPS (1½ TO 2 POUNDS TOTAL), TRIMMED

1 TABLESPOON CHOPPED FRESH MINT

1. Preheat the oven to 375°F.

2. In a medium saucepan, heat 2 teaspoons of the olive oil over medium heat. Add the garlic and cook, stirring constantly, for 1 minute. Add the peas, water, and ¼ teaspoon of the salt and bring to a boil. Lower the heat, cover, and simmer for 5 minutes. Remove the pan from the heat.

3. Sprinkle both sides of the lamb chops with the remaining ½ teaspoon of salt and the pepper. In a large oven-safe skillet, heat the remaining 2 teaspoons olive oil over medium-high heat. Add the lamb chops and cook until browned on the bottom, about 2 minutes. Turn the chops over and transfer the skillet to the oven.

4. Bake until the desired degree of doneness has been achieved, 8 to 12 minutes for medium-rare.

5. While the meat is in the oven, place the pea mixture in a food processor, add the mint, and pulse to a coarse puree. If the mixture is too thick, add a bit more water, 1 tablespoon at a time, to thin it.

6. Spoon some of the puree onto each of 4 serving plates and top each with 2 lamb chops. Serve immediately.

CHAPTER 10

Desserts

Honey Custard with Tropical Fruit

SERVES 4

Honey has a lower glycemic index than sugar, plus it has lots of essential minerals, antibacterial properties, and a distinctive, rich flavor, making it a great substitute for refined sugar. Here honey flavors a smooth, creamy custard made with low-fat milk. A tumble of tropical fruits finishes off the dish with bright colors and lots of sweet, fruity flavor.

3 LARGE EGGS

¼ CUP HONEY

1 TEASPOON PURE VANILLA EXTRACT

⅛ TEASPOON SALT

2 CUPS 1 PERCENT MILK

1½ CUPS DICED PINEAPPLE (FRESH OR CANNED, DRAINED)

3 KIWIS, PEELED AND DICED

1 RIPE MANGO, PEELED AND DICED

2 BANANAS, DICED

1. Preheat the oven to 300°F and place four 6-ounce ramekins in a 2-inch-deep baking pan.

2. In a large bowl, beat the eggs. Add the honey, vanilla, and salt and beat until incorporated. In a small saucepan, heat the milk over medium high-heat, stirring constantly, until it's hot but not boiling. Whisking constantly, slowly add the hot milk to the egg mixture and mix until incorporated.

3. Ladle the custard mixture into the ramekins, dividing evenly. Pour hot water into the pan, being careful not to splash any into the custard, so that it comes about halfway up the sides of the ramekins. Bake until the custard is fully set, about 1 hour. Set the ramekins on a wire rack to cool to room temperature.

4. While the custard is cooling, combine the pineapple, kiwi, mango, and banana in a large bowl and toss to mix.

5. Run a knife around the edge of each custard and then invert it onto a dessert plate. Top with a generous scoop of fruit and serve.

Peach-Blueberry Crisp

SERVES 6

Fruit crisps are a great way to satisfy a craving for pie, without the bother of making a pastry crust (or the extra fat, calories, and refined carb it adds). This peach-blueberry version is great to make in the height of summer when stone fruits and berries are at their peak, but you can vary it to include any fruits that are in season. Try apples and blackberries, pears and cranberries, strawberries and rhubarb, or whatever combination appeals to you.

FILLING:

2 TABLESPOONS BROWN SUGAR

1½ TABLESPOONS CORNSTARCH

1 TABLESPOON FRESHLY SQUEEZED LEMON JUICE

1 TEASPOON LEMON ZEST

1 TEASPOON GROUND CINNAMON

2 CUPS BLUEBERRIES

2 CUPS CHOPPED PEELED PEACHES

TOPPING:

¼ CUP WHOLE-WHEAT FLOUR

¼ CUP OLD-FASHIONED OATS

3 TABLESPOONS BROWN SUGAR

3 TABLESPOONS UNSALTED BUTTER, CUT INTO SMALL PIECES

¼ CUP SLICED ALMONDS

1. Preheat the oven to 350°F.

2. In a large bowl, combine the brown sugar, cornstarch, lemon juice, lemon zest, and cinnamon. Add the blueberries and peaches and toss gently to coat. Transfer to a large baking dish.

3. In a medium bowl, combine the flour, oats, and brown sugar. Cut the butter into the dry ingredients with a fork or pastry cutter until the mixture resembles coarse crumbs. Stir in the almonds. Sprinkle the topping evenly over the fruit.

4. Bake the crisp until the topping is browned and the filling is bubbly, about 10 minutes. Serve immediately.

Apricot Filo Tart

SERVES 4

Filo dough is that tissue-thin Greek pastry that's used to make both sweet and savory tarts and filled pies. You can usually find whole-wheat filo dough at natural foods stores like Whole Food Market, but if it's not available, substitute regular filo dough. Either way, this flaky, fruit-filled tart has far less fat and calories than one made with a traditional pastry crust.

3 LARGE (9-BY-14-INCH) SHEETS WHOLE-WHEAT FILO DOUGH,
    AT ROOM TEMPERATURE

2 TABLESPOONS UNSALTED BUTTER, MELTED

3 TABLESPOONS APRICOT JAM, WARMED IN THE MICROWAVE OR A
    SAUCEPAN ON THE STOVE

8 TO 10 RIPE APRICOTS, SLICED

1. Preheat the oven to 400°F.

2. Lay a large piece of parchment paper on your work surface. Lay 1 sheet of filo dough on the parchment paper and brush it with butter. Top with a second piece of filo. Brush with butter again. Lay the third piece of filo on top and brush once more with butter. Fold the layered filo dough in half so that you have a 9-by-7-inch rectangle that is 6 layers thick. Fold up the edges of the pastry on all four sides to create a 1-inch raised border. Spread the warmed jam on the tart, covering the entire surface inside the border. Slide the parchment and crust onto a baking sheet and bake for 5 minutes.

3. Remove the crust from the oven and arrange the apricots over the tart in a decorative pattern. If you have any butter left, brush it over the apricots. Return the tart to the oven and bake until the pastry is crisp and golden brown, about 20 minutes. Serve warm or at room temperature.

Chocolate Chip Cookies

MAKES ABOUT 2½ DOZEN COOKIES

This classic cookie, a time-honored favorite, gets a nutrition boost from a combination of fiber- and nutrient-rich whole-wheat flour, protein-heavy almond flour, and nutritious flaxseed meal. Plus it has much less sugar than traditional recipes. On top of all that, these cookies are scrumptious. Serve them with a glass of cold milk and relive those carefree days of childhood without a hint of guilt.

COOKING SPRAY

1 CUP WHOLE-WHEAT FLOUR

¾ CUP ALMOND FLOUR

2 TABLESPOONS FLAXSEED MEAL

½ TEASPOON BAKING POWDER

½ TEASPOON SALT

¼ CUP UNSALTED BUTTER, AT ROOM TEMPERATURE

¼ CUP GRANULATED SUGAR

¼ CUP PACKED BROWN SUGAR

¼ CUP COCONUT OR CANOLA OIL

1 LARGE EGG, LIGHTLY BEATEN

1 TEASPOON PURE VANILLA EXTRACT

1 CUP SEMISWEET CHOCOLATE CHIPS

1. Preheat the oven to 350°F and spray two large baking sheets with cooking spray.

2. In a medium bowl, combine the whole-wheat flour, almond flour, flaxseed meal, baking powder, and salt.

3. In a large bowl, cream together the butter and both sugars using an electric mixer. Add the coconut or canola oil, egg, and vanilla and mix to combine.

4. Add the flour mixture to the wet ingredients and mix on low speed until incorporated. Stir in the chocolate chips.

5. Drop the dough by the heaping teaspoonful onto the prepared baking sheets, leaving at least 1 inch in between for spreading. Bake until golden brown around the edges, about 10 minutes. Let the cookies cool on the baking sheets for a couple of minutes and then transfer to a wire rack to cool completely. Serve warm or at room temperature.

Almond-Sesame Crunch Cookies

These crispy, crunchy cookies are packed with all the goodness of sesame seeds, which contain omega-3 fatty acids and phytonutrients in addition to their rich, nutty flavor.

¾ CUP WHOLE-WHEAT FLOUR

¾ CUP ALMOND FLOUR

1½ TABLESPOONS CORNSTARCH

1 TEASPOON BAKING POWDER

½ TEASPOON BAKING SODA

¼ TEASPOON SALT

1 CUP PACKED BROWN SUGAR

⅓ CUP TAHINI

2 TABLESPOONS TOASTED SESAME OIL

1 TABLESPOON LIGHT CORN SYRUP

2 TEASPOONS PURE VANILLA EXTRACT

1 LARGE EGG

2 TABLESPOONS GRANULATED SUGAR

1. Preheat the oven to 375°F and line two large baking sheets with parchment paper.

2. In a medium bowl, combine the whole-wheat flour, almond flour, cornstarch, baking powder, baking soda, and salt.

3. In a large mixing bowl, cream together the brown sugar, tahini, and sesame oil with an electric mixer set on medium speed. Add the syrup, vanilla, and egg and beat to incorporate. With the mixer on low, add the flour mixture and mix to incorporate.

4. Put the granulated sugar in a shallow bowl.

5. Shape the dough into 1-inch balls.

6. Roll the balls of dough in the granulated sugar and then place them on the prepared baking sheets, about 2 inches apart, flattening the dough balls with the palm of your hand.

7. Bake until lightly browned, about 10 minutes. Let the cookies cool on the baking sheets for a couple of minutes and then transfer to a wire rack to cool completely. Serve warm or at room temperature.

Oatmeal-Raisin-Nut Cookies

MAKES ABOUT 2 DOZEN COOKIES

These wonderfully chewy cookies get extra fiber and nutrients from wheat germ and flaxseed meal. This recipe also substitutes whole-wheat flour for most of the white flour found in most cookie recipes, and reduces the sugar by adding unsweetened applesauce and lots of plump, sweet raisins.

½ CUP WHOLE-WHEAT FLOUR

¼ CUP ALL-PURPOSE FLOUR

2 TABLESPOONS WHEAT GERM

2 TABLESPOONS FLAXSEED MEAL

½ TEASPOON BAKING SODA

½ TEASPOON GROUND CINNAMON

¼ TEASPOON SALT

½ CUP UNSALTED BUTTER, AT ROOM TEMPERATURE

½ CUP PACKED BROWN SUGAR

¼ CUP UNSWEETENED APPLESAUCE

1 LARGE EGG

½ TEASPOON PURE VANILLA EXTRACT

1½ CUPS OLD-FASHIONED ROLLED OATS

¾ CUP RAISINS

½ CUP WALNUTS, CHOPPED

1. Preheat the oven to 350°F and line two large baking sheets with parchment paper.

2. In a medium bowl, combine both flours, the wheat germ, flaxseed meal, baking soda, cinnamon, and salt.

3. In a large bowl, using an electric mixer, cream the butter and brown sugar together. Add the applesauce, egg, and vanilla and mix to incorporate.

4. Add the dry mixture to the wet mixture and beat to combine. Stir in the oats, raisins, and walnuts.

5. Scoop the dough onto the prepared baking sheets by the rounded table-spoonful, spacing them about 2 inches apart. Bake until they are beginning to turn golden brown, 10 to 12 minutes. Let the cookies cool on the baking sheets for a few minutes before transferring them to a wire rack to cool completely. Serve warm or at room temperature.

Lemon–Poppy Seed Greek Yogurt Cake

SERVES 8 TO 10

Greek yogurt keeps this cake super moist, while poppy seeds add healthy monoun-saturated fats, minerals, and antioxidants. Using almond flour instead of wheat flour gives it extra protein and fiber. With a bright lemony tang, this light cake is the perfect thing to satisfy a sweet tooth without sending your diet off the rails.

COOKING SPRAY

2½ CUPS ALMOND FLOUR

2 TEASPOONS BAKING POWDER

2 CUPS PLAIN LOW-FAT GREEK YOGURT

4 LARGE EGGS, SEPARATED

½ CUP HONEY

⅓ CUP FRESHLY SQUEEZED LEMON JUICE

1 TABLESPOON LEMON ZEST

2 TEASPOONS PURE VANILLA EXTRACT

1. Preheat the oven to 350°F. Spray a 9-inch square cake pan with cooking spray and line it with parchment paper.

2. In a large bowl, stir together the almond flour and baking powder. Add the yogurt, egg yolks, honey, lemon juice, lemon zest, and vanilla and stir to incorporate.

3. In a separate large bowl, beat the egg whites with an electric mixer set on medium until soft peaks form. Gently fold the whites into the batter.

4. Transfer the batter to the prepared cake pan and bake for 40 minutes. Cover the cake with foil and continue to bake until a toothpick inserted into the center comes out clean, about 20 minutes more.

5. Let the cake cool in the pan on a wire rack for about 10 minutes. Invert the cake onto the rack and cool to room temperature before serving.

Coconut-Frosted Carrot Cake

A cake that's packed with carrots has to be healthy, right? While that may not always be true, in this case you're in luck! This gluten-free, dairy-free cake is studded with sweet raisins, nutty walnuts, and, of course, plenty of shredded carrots. Sweetened with just a touch of honey or agave nectar and spiced with cinnamon and nutmeg, this healthy cake recipe is a winner.

CAKE:

COOKING SPRAY

3 CUPS ALMOND FLOUR

1 TEASPOON SALT

1 TEASPOON BAKING SODA

1 TEASPOON GROUND CINNAMON

1 TEASPOON GROUND NUTMEG

5 LARGE EGGS

½ CUP HONEY OR AGAVE NECTAR

¼ CUP COCONUT OR CANOLA OIL

3 CUPS GRATED CARROTS

1 CUP RAISINS

1 CUP CHOPPED WALNUTS

FROSTING:

1 CUP UNSWEETENED COCONUT CREAM,* CHILLED IN THE
   REFRIGERATOR OVERNIGHT

1 TABLESPOON HONEY OR AGAVE NECTAR

½ TEASPOON PURE VANILLA EXTRACT

½ CUP UNSWEETENED FLAKED COCONUT, TOASTED (OPTIONAL)

1. Preheat the oven to 350°F and spray two 9-inch round cake pans with cooking spray.

continued ▶

2. In a large bowl, combine the almond flour, salt, baking soda, cinnamon, and nutmeg.

3. In a medium bowl, whisk together the eggs, honey or agave nectar, and oil. Add the carrots, raisins, and walnuts and stir to combine.

4. Mix the wet ingredients into the dry ingredients until incorporated.

5. Transfer the batter to the prepared baking pans, dividing evenly, and bake until a toothpick inserted into the center comes out clean, 30 to 35 minutes.

6. Let the cakes cool in the pans for about 5 minutes, then invert onto a wire rack to cool completely.

7. To make the frosting, place the coconut cream in a large mixing bowl and beat with an electric mixer set on high until it's light and fluffy, about 5 minutes. Add the honey or agave nectar and the vanilla and beat to incorporate.

8. To assemble the cake, place the first layer, bottom side down, on a cake plate. Use a spatula to spread the frosting to cover the top of the layer. Place the second layer on top of the first, top side down. Spread on more frosting to cover the top and sides of the cake. Top with the toasted coconut flakes, if using.

*If you can't find coconut cream, substitute a 15-ounce can of full-fat coconut milk. After chilling the can overnight, flip it over, open it, and then pour off the thin liquid, retaining only the thick cream underneath it.

The Healthiest Brownies

MAKES 12 BROWNIES

Think a brownie can't be both healthy and delicious? Well, think again. These rich, chocolaty brownies contain a secret source of protein and fiber: black beans! The beans also add moisture, which reduces the amount of added fat. And the sugar is kept to a minimum, too. Try baking these in a mini muffin tin for portion-controlled treats perfect for tucking into a lunchbox.

COOKING SPRAY

1 (15-OUNCE) CAN BLACK BEANS, RINSED AND DRAINED

½ CUP OLD-FASHIONED ROLLED OATS

½ CUP SUGAR

¼ CUP COCONUT OR CANOLA OIL

2 TABLESPOONS UNSWEETENED COCOA POWDER

2 TEASPOONS PURE VANILLA EXTRACT

½ TEASPOON BAKING POWDER

¼ TEASPOON SALT

½ CUP SEMISWEET CHOCOLATE CHIPS

⅓ CUP CHOPPED WALNUTS, PECANS, ALMONDS, OR
    HAZELNUTS (OPTIONAL)

1. Preheat the oven to 350°F and spray an 8-inch square baking pan with cooking spray.

2. Combine the beans, oats, sugar, oil, cocoa powder, vanilla, baking powder, and salt in a food processor and process until smooth. Stir in the chocolate chips and nuts, if using.

3. Transfer the batter to the prepared baking pan and bake until the edges are dry and beginning to pull away from the pan, 16 to 18 minutes. Let cool in the pan for at least 10 minutes before cutting and serving.

Luscious Chocolate Pudding

SERVES 6

Once you taste this pudding, you'll have a hard time believing that it's dairy-free—even if you made it yourself. It gets its luxurious creaminess from avocado, which contains healthy monounsaturated fat. And its sweetness comes from a dash of maple syrup and a ripe banana instead of refined sugar. Serve this pudding very cold in small custard bowls or teacups for a simple yet elegant dessert.

2 HASS AVOCADOS, PEELED AND CUT INTO CHUNKS

1 BANANA, CUT INTO CHUNKS

1 CUP UNSWEETENED ALMOND MILK

¼ CUP UNSWEETENED COCOA POWDER

2 TABLESPOONS PURE MAPLE SYRUP

1 TEASPOON PURE VANILLA EXTRACT

½ TEASPOON GROUND CINNAMON

1. Place the avocado, banana, almond milk, cocoa powder, maple syrup, vanilla, and cinnamon in a blender and process until very smooth.

2. Transfer the mixture to a bowl, or to six 6-ounce ramekins or custard cups, cover, and chill in the refrigerator for at least 4 hours. Serve cold.

Index

CPSIA information can be obtained
at www.ICGtesting.com
Printed in the USA
LVHW081715230119
604976LV00029B/668/P

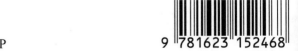

9 781623 152468